Integrative Anatomy Review

FIRST EDITION

Robert Tyler Morris

Missouri State University

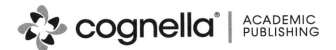 cognella® | ACADEMIC PUBLISHING

Bassim Hamadeh, CEO and Publisher

Angela Schultz, Acquisitions Editor

Michelle Piehl, Project Edito

Berenice Quirino, Associate Production Editor

Jess Estrella, Senior Graphic Designer r

Trey Soto, Licensing Associate

Don Kesner, Interior Designer

Natalie Piccotti, Senior Marketing Manager

Kassie Graves, Director of Acquisitions and Sales

Jamie Giganti, Senior Managing Editor

Cover image copyright © 2013 iStockphoto LP/MedicalArtInc

Printed in the United States of America.

ISBN: 978-1-5165-0243-1 (pbk) / 978-1-5165-0244-8 (br)

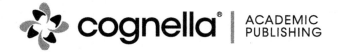

cognella® | ACADEMIC PUBLISHING

Integrative
Anatomy Review

CONTENTS

Preface

> "I hear and I forget. I see and I remember.
> I do and I understand."
> —A 2000-year-old proverb

Anatomy is a keystone for understanding human health and disease. In collaboration with 4D Anatomy (www.4Danatomy.com), *Integrative Anatomy Review* presents high yield information while creating a dynamic working model for the student. This unique approach includes (1) the discussion of the essential concepts, (2) the visualization of select cadaver views, and (3) the connection to important **clinical considerations (blue).** A variety of **Concept Maps (CM)** and **Synthesis Exercises (EX)** will also assist students with integrating the challenging concepts. Based upon educational research (Blunt JR, Karpicke JD, J Educational Psychology, 2014), retrieval-based concept mapping provides an efficient and interactive technique for learning. *Integrative Anatomy Review* is the first comprehensive anatomy textbook to use this mechanism of learning. Furthermore, access to 4D Anatomy provides the student with an extensive online library of prosected cadaver images.

HOW TO USE THIS TEXTBOOK:

Target audience For individual students, small groups, or classrooms.

What settings are best for use of this textbook? For lecture, laboratory, or review outside of the classroom

What scholastic groups can use this textbook? For undergraduate and health professional students

What supplemental materials are recommended to maximize learning with this textbook? A large ink board and various color markers, or paper and colored pencils

CHAPTER 1
Back

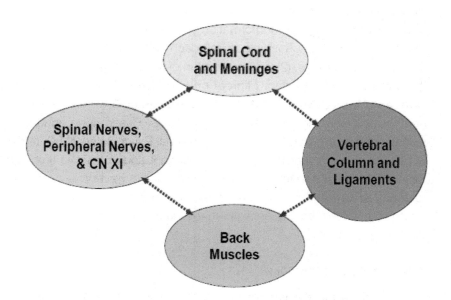

I. Vertebral Column and Ligaments

Overview of topics for this section:

- Surface anatomy of the back
- Structural support for the back
- Upper body weight transfer to lower limbs
- Curvature of the vertebral column
- Osteoporosis, excessive lumbar lordosis, scoliosis
- Ligaments preventing hyperextension and hyperflexion
- Intervertebral discs and herniation

What surface anatomy landmarks can be observed on the back?

The **vertebra prominens** is a spinous process of cervical vertebra-7 (C7) and results in a bony protuberance which can be palpated at the base of the posterior neck. The **posterior median furrow** is a midline depression of the back (particularly observed in a fit person) due to the impression of the trapezius muscle and deep back muscles. Inferiorly, the (posterior superior iliac spine **[PSIS]**, or Venusian Dimples) represent bilateral depressions in the lower back at the sacrum level 2 (S2) (also particularly observed in a fit person). The borders of the trapezius and latissimus dorsi muscles form the **triangle of auscultation**, a relatively unexposed region allowing a clinician to listen to breathing or heart beat via a stethoscope.

What is the main source of structural support for the upper body? How is it characterized in the neck, upper back, and lower back? What skeletal features help translate specific movements in the head, cervical, thoracic, and lumbar regions?

Osteology of the vertebral column — The vertebral column is created by a series of bones called vertebrae derived from embryonic mesoderm tissue. In addition to interlocking joints of adjacent vertebrae, stability is reinforced by ligaments and muscles (described later). Some functions of the vertebral column are to maintain posture, support weight of the body, transmit body weight to lower limbs, assist with locomotion, provide a rigid but flexible axis for the body and head, and protect the spinal cord and nerve roots. A specific number of vertebra exist in each of five regions within the vertebral column: seven cervical vertebrae (C1–C7), 12 thoracic vertebrae (T1–T12), five lumbar vertebrae (L1–L5), five fused sacral vertebrae (S1–S5), and a variable number of fused coccygeal vertebrae (remnants of a tailbone).

A typical vertebra includes the following features: an anterior vertebral body composed of spongy bone (central) and a thin layer of peripheral compact bone; and a vertebral arch, which surrounds the vertebral foramen and houses the spinal cord. The vertebral arch is produced by a pedicle (a structure that connects an organ to the body) and lamina (which forms the posterior aspect of the arch). A bony protuberance directed posteriorly, called the spinous process, is a common site of muscle attachment. Similarly, right and left transverse processes project bilaterally from the vertebral arch. The intervertebral foramen is lateral opening between two adjacent vertebrae; spinal nerves exit from the spinal cord here. Articular processes extend superiorly and inferiorly. Facets (flat surfaces) of each process allow articulation of vertebral joints. For example, the inferior process from adjacent vertebrae above and the superior process from below articulate to form zygapophysial (facet) joints.

The five regions of the vertebral column (C, T, L, S, and coccygeal) have modifications that promote unique functions. In the cervical region (C1–C7), no true vertebral bodies exist. However, a unique transverse foramina is present, through which the bilateral vertebral artery passes to the skull. The atlas, or C1 vertebra (holding the earth), articulates with the occipital condyles of the skull via the atlanto-occipital joint, allowing for a variety of movements (rotation, flexion, extension). The axis, or C2 vertebra, which assists in rotation, includes an anterosuperior protuberance called the dens, which articulates with C1 to further promote rotation of the skull. Also, the atlanto-axial joint is formed between C1 and C2 between the articular processes of each. Anteriorly placed ligaments between the occipital bone, C1, and C2, called cruciate ligaments (crossing pattern) help stabilize this region. Thoracic vertebrae (T1–T12) have relatively long spinous processes. The articular facets in this region project anteriorly and posteriorly within the coronal plane. Thus, rotational movements are possible (twisting of torso), while little flexion and extension occurs. In addition to facet joints, the thoracic vertebrae possess facets for articulation with the ribs. The vertebral bodies have both a superior and inferior costal facet for the head of the rib. This creates a **costovertebral joint**. The transverse process has a costal facet for the tubercle of the rib which creates a **costotransverse joint**. Functionally, the costovertebral and costotransverse joints allow the rib an axis of movement during deep respiratory movements (see Thorax Unit). In contrast, lumbar vertebrae (L1–L5) have relatively large vertebral bodies and possess articular facets that face in a lateral direction within the sagittal plane. As a result, the lumbar region primarily allows flexion and extension of the torso with little to no rotational movements. The sacrum (S1–S5) includes 5 fused vertebrae, beginning superiorly with the sacral base. The sacral promontory is a distinct anterior ridge of the first sacral body. Bilateral wing-like edges of the sacrum are called the **alae**. The sacral canal is a posterior passageway for the remaining inferior spinal nerves of the cauda equina (described later). Finally, the sacral foramina are passageways for spinal nerves, which are segmented and bilateral. Anterior and posterior rami from each spinal nerve exit from the sacral foramina in their respective directions.

Clinical Consideration – How is upper body weight transferred to the lower limbs and what type of dysfunction can occur at this joint?

The bilateral articular surface of the sacrum joins with the articular surface of the ileum. This site of articulation, or sacroiliac joint (SI), helps transfer weight from the upper body to the lower limbs. A variety of ligaments help stabilize the sacrum during transmission of force (e.g., running, jumping). Cartilage lines the articular surfaces to reduce friction between these bones. However, when the cartilage wears down, a patient can experience pain and limited movement at this joint. This condition of the SI joint, known as degenerative arthritis, or osteoarthritis, can occur due to aging, overuse, and obesity.

What accounts for curvature of the vertebral column in very specific regions? What are these curvatures called?

The shape of the vertebral column begins as a concave, anterior C-shape in utero. The primary curvature, called the **kyphoses**, occurs in the thoracic and sacral regions. Concave, posterior secondary curvatures, called lordosis, develop later in life. As infants attain muscular control of the head and neck, a cervical **lordosis** develops. The act of standing and subsequent support of the upper body initiates a lumbar lordosis. Taken together, the adult vertebral column is not straight, but curved in specific regions.

Clinical Consideration – What clinical conditions can affect the shape of the vertebral column?

Osteoporosis, or bone degeneration, is commonly facilitated by aging. Fragile, weak bones can lead to increased risk of fracture. Excessive thoracic kyphosis (i.e hump back) may occur in the presence of weakened vertebrae. Alternatively, excessive lumbar lordosis (i.e., hollow back) may ensue temporarily during pregnancy. Abnormal lateral curvature of spine, called scoliosis, may occur due to unequal lower limb lengths or poor develop of the intrinsic back muscles.

What ligaments of the back prevent hyperextension? Hyperflexion? Identify a type of event which may damage these ligaments.

The **anterior longitudinal ligament** is a broad ligament, located anterior to the vertebral bodies, that limits hyperextension of the vertebral column. Similarly, the narrower **posterior longitudinal ligament**, located posterior to the vertebral bodies within the vertebral canal, limits hyperflexion. The **nuchal ligament** attaches to the spinous processes of cervical vertebrae and is a good attachment site for muscles. The **ligamentum flava** spans adjacent lamina of the vertebrae. Automobile accidents and associated "whiplash" of the head and neck are risk factors for ligament damage or tearing in the cervical region.

What is an Intervertebral Disc (IV)?

Intervertebral (IV) discs found between vertebral bodies serve as a cushioning system, buffering forces generated through the vertebral column. The IV discs include an outer portion, called the annulus fibrosus (AF) made of fibrocartilage, and a gelatinous inner portion somewhat like a water balloon, called a nucleus pulposus (NP), made of reticular and collagenous fibers. Importantly, movements of the thorax and lumbar region can compress the nucleus pulposus. For example, flexion of the torso promotes a posterior movement of NP due to the anterior compression of the vertebral bodies. However, extension of the torso can move the NP anteriorly, and lateral flexion can facilitate movement of the NP to the contralateral side.

Clinical Consideration - What is a herniated or slipped intervertebral disc? What risk factors contribute to this? How does this impact adjacent spinal nerves? How do IV discs frequently herniate in the posterior-lateral direction?

A herniated IV disc can occur due to excessive compression or force within the vertebral column. For example, lifting a heavy object (e.g., a couch) can compress the anterior aspect of the vertebral bodies.

Consequently, the NP may exit the AF posteriolaterally and compress (or pinch) a local spinal nerve. Sciatica (pain in lower back, hip, and thigh) can be caused by herniation any of the L5–S1 discs and subsequent compression of local spinal nerves. The anatomy of the IV foramen spares the spinal nerve of the same segment from compression, because the nerve exits superior to the herniation. However, the next spinal nerve is typically affected.

See CM 1-1A, 1-1B, 1-1C, 1-1D, 1-1E, and 1-1F for Review.

CM 1-1A

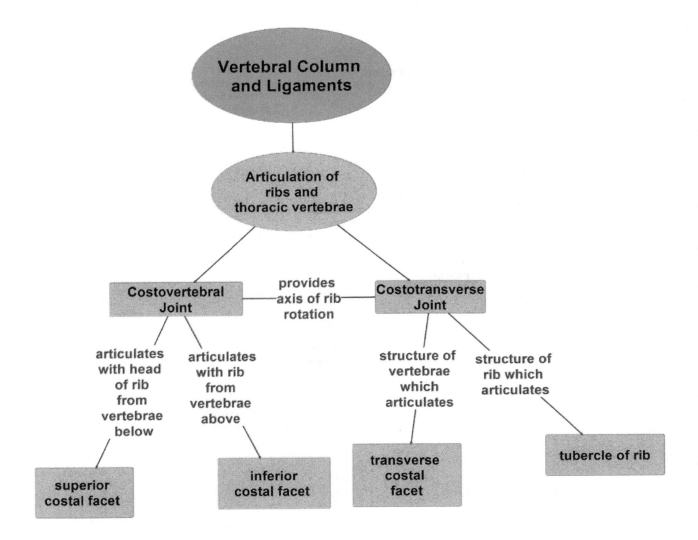

CM 1-1B

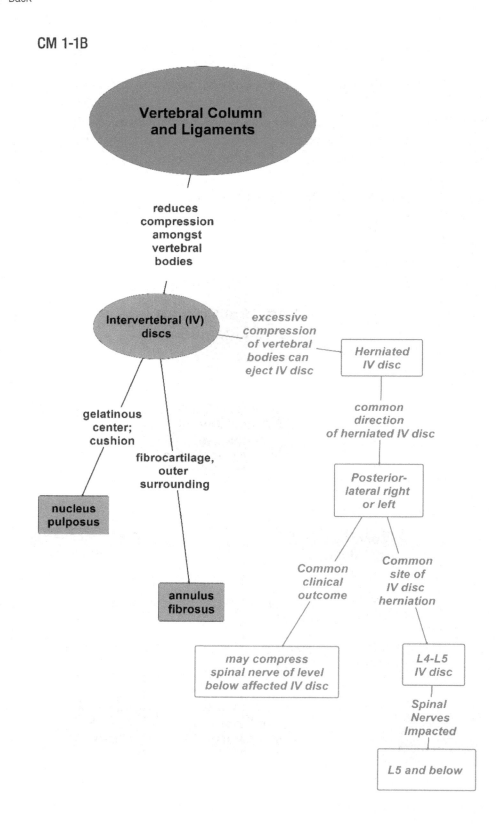

CM 1-1C

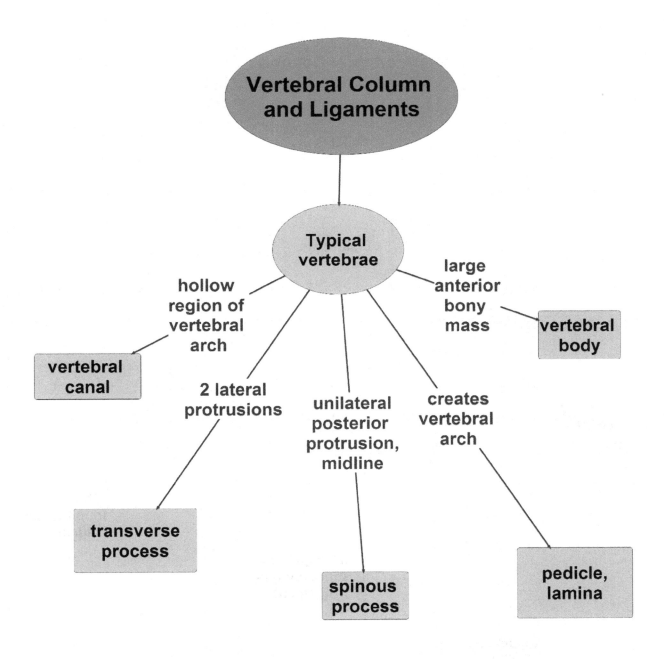

CHAPTER 1

CM 1-1D

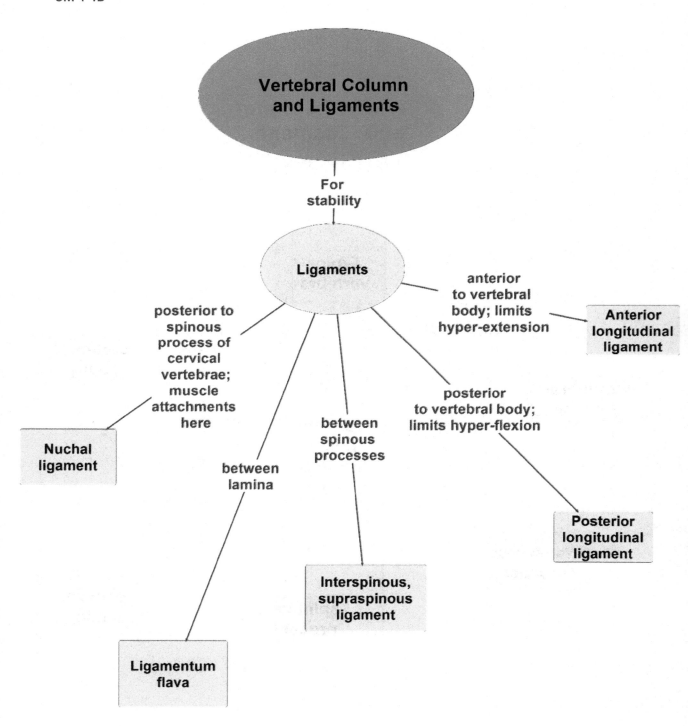

CM 1-1E

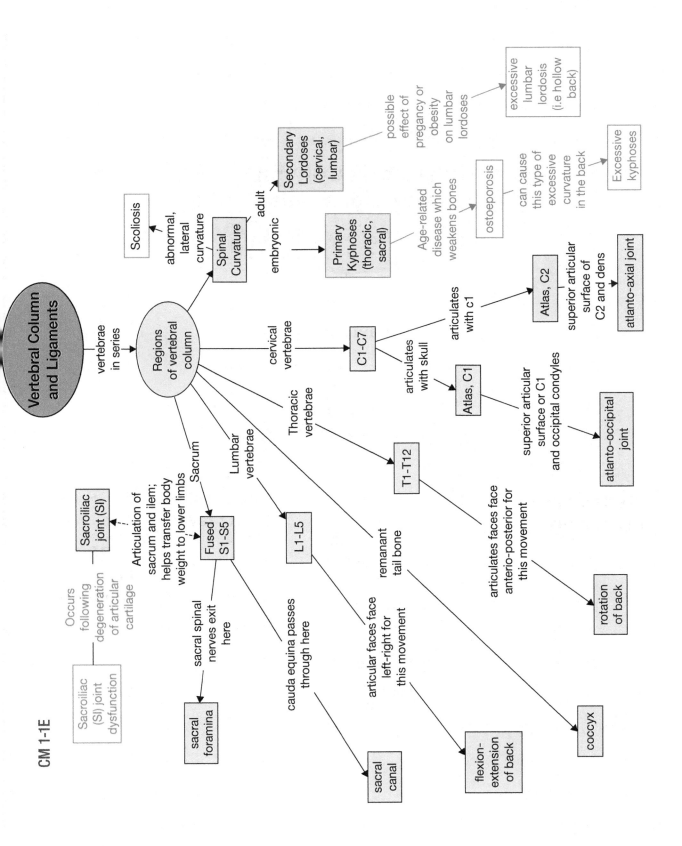

CM 1-1F

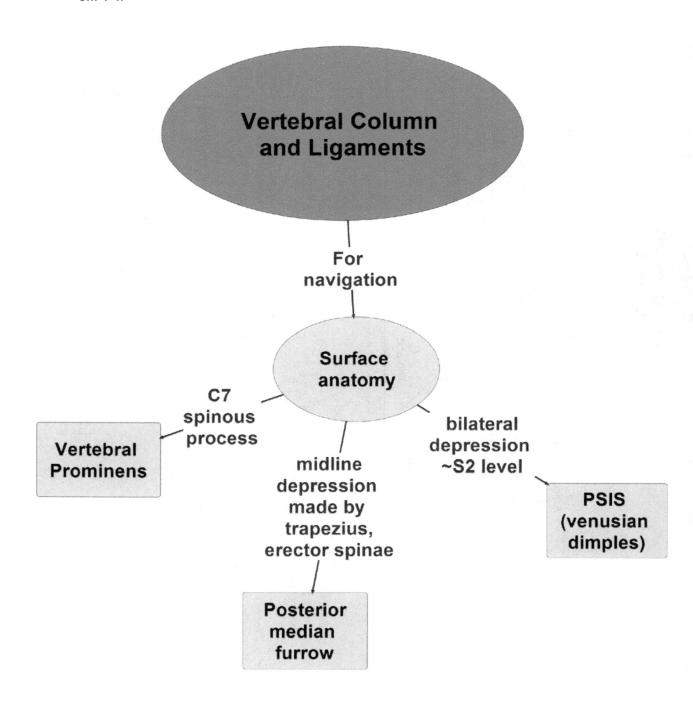

Synthesis Exercise: Create a concept map using items from EXERCISE 1-1A, 1-1B, 1-1C, 1-1D, 1-1E, and 1-1F.

Exercise 1-1A

Primary Category	Secondary Category	Continuations
Vertebral Column and Ligaments	Articulations of ribs and thoracic vertebrae	Costotransverse Joint Costovertebral Joint Transverse Costal Facet Tubercle of rib Inferior costal facet Superior costal facet

Exercise 1-1B

Primary Category	Secondary Category	Continuations	Clinical Considerations
Vertebral Column and Ligaments	IV discs	Nucleus pulposus Annulus fibrosus	Herniated IV disc L4-L5 IV disc Posterior lateral left or right Compression of spinal nerve

Exercise 1-1C

Primary Category	Secondary Category	Continuations
Vertebral Column and Ligaments	Typical vertebrae	Vertebral canal Vertebral body Pedicle Lamina Spinous process Transverse process

Exercise 1-1D

Primary Category	Secondary Category	Continuations
Vertebral Column and Ligaments	Ligaments	Anterior longitudinal ligament
		Posterior longitudinal ligament
		Interspinous ligament
		Supraspinous ligament
		Ligamentum flava
		Nuchal ligament

Exercise 1-1E

Primary Category	Secondary Category	Continuations	Clinical Considerations
Vertebral Column and Ligaments	Regions of the vertebral column	Spinal curvature	SI joint dysfunction
		Primary and Secondary Lordoses	Scoliosis
		Primary and Secondary Kyphoses	Osteoporosis
		C1-C7 vertebrae	Excessive kyphosis
		Atlas	Excessive lordosis
		Axis	
		Atlanto-axial joint	
		Atlanto-occipital joint	
		T1-T12 vertebrae	
		Rotation of back	
		L1-L5 vertebrae	
		Vertebral Prominens	
		S1-S5 vertrbrae	
		Sacrum	
		Sacral canal	
		Sacral foramina	
		Coccyx	
		Flexion-extension of back	
		Sacroilliac joint	
		PSIS	
		Posterior Median Furrow	
		Vertebral Prominens	

Exercise 1-1F

Primary Category	Secondary Category	Continuations
Vertebral Column and Ligaments	Surface anatomy	PSIS Posterior Median Furrow Vertebral Prominens

II. Back Muscles

Overview of topics for this section:

- Superficial back anatomy, including muscles, key attachments, innervation, and actions
- Spinal accessory nerve (CN XI) palsy
- Thoracodorsal nerve damage
- Intermediate neck, including muscles, key attachments, innervation, and actions
- Deep and very deep back, including muscles, key attachments, innervation, and actions
- Suboccipital triangle

What single muscle can elevate, retract, and depress the scapula? Explain how one muscle can contribute to three different types of movements?

Muscles and Fasciae of The Superficial Back

1   trapezius

2   latissimus dorsi

3   thoracolumbar fascia

The **trapezius** muscle has three divisions with variation in muscle fibers attachments, each of which has different functionality **(see figure 1-1)**.

Figure 1-1

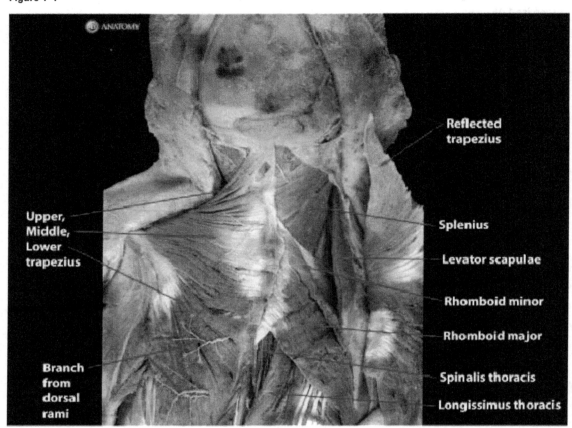

Reflected trapezius

Upper, Middle, Lower trapezius

Splenius

Levator scapulae

Rhomboid minor

Rhomboid major

Branch from dorsal rami

Spinalis thoracis

Longissimus thoracis

Superiorly, the upper division (descending trapezius) attaches at the superior nuchal line, nuchal ligament, acromion, and lateral **clavicles**. The middle division attaches at the spinous processes of vertebrae and scapular spine. Inferiorly, the lower division (ascending trapezius) has similar attachments as the middle division. The middle and lower divisions attach within a range of C7–T12 medially. The **spinal accessory nerve** (CN XI) innervates the trapezius and its arterial supply is the **transverse cervical artery**. Contraction of the upper division of the trapezius leads to upward rotation and elevation of the **scapula**; contraction of the middle division causes retraction of the scapula; and contraction of the inferior division results in depression of the scapula. Injury to CN XI can lead to trapezius dysfunction, such as inability to elevate the shoulders or a drooping shoulder on the ipsilateral side (*side of injury*). To test trapezius function, observe movements of the scapula (*shoulder*) as described above upon contraction.

Clinical Consideration — What are the effects of spinal accessory nerve (CN XI) palsy or injury?

Damage or injury to the spinal accessory nerve can occur during trauma, lymph node biopsy, or jugular vein cannulation. Symptoms include atrophy of the trapezius muscle, a drooping shoulder, and shoulder pain.

Which single muscle of the back functions to adduct, internally rotate, and extend the upper limb?

The **latissimus dorsi** muscle is a superficial muscle located on the lateral and mid-back. It has several proximal attachments along the spinous processes of thoracic T7–L5, including the thoracolumbar fascia, iliac crest, inferior three or four ribs, and the inferior angle of scapula. The distal attachment occurs at the floor of intertubercular groove of the **humerus**. During contraction, the upper limb can be adducted, extended, or internally rotated. The arterial supply is the thoracodorsal branch of the subscapular artery. Innervation to the latissimus dorsi is via the thoracodorsal nerve from the brachial plexus. A thick investing membrane, called the **thoracolumbar fascia**, covers the muscles of the superficial and deep lower back,. Weakness of adduction or extension at the shoulder may indicate a an ipsilateral injury. To test latissimus dorsi function, a clinician may provide resistance against adduction of the upper limb.

Clinical Consideration — What are the effects of thoracodorsal nerve damage? What alternative muscles may help compensate in this setting?

Patients with thoracodorsal nerve injury may experience weakened ability to adduct the upper limb against resistance. For example, pull ups or swimming (e.g., breast stroke) may be difficult on the side of injury. However, other muscles can compensate for the lack of latissimus dorsi function, such as the posterior deltoid and teres major.

What additional back muscles act on the scapula?

Muscles of The Intermediate Back

1   rhomboid major & minor
2   levator scapulae
3   serratus posterior inferior, serratus posterior superior

The **rhomboid** muscle has a major and minor division (**see figure 1-1**). The major is more inferior and larger compared to the minor. These attach from C7–T5 spinous process to the medial border of the scapula, and due to the oblique angle of the muscle fibers, the scapula is both retracted and the glenoid head is rotated inferiorly during contraction. The dorsal scapular nerve and artery, innervate and supply blood, respectively.

The **levator scapulae** muscle has several "ribbon like" muscle bellies (**see figure 1-1)**. They elevate the scapula and also rotate the glenoid head inferiorly during contraction. Attachments include C1–C4 transverse processes and the superior angle of the scapula. The dorsal scapular nerve innervates, and the dorsal scapular artery supplies blood to the levator scapulae.

What muscle group communicates the amount of expansion and compression in the thoracic wall to the CNS?

The serratus posterior superior (deep to the rhomboids) **(see figure 1-2)** and serratus posterior inferior (deep to the latissimus dorsi) are located in an intermediate plane. These relatively thin muscles likely do not generate significant amounts of force, but are primarily involved with proprioception of the thoracic wall during forced respiration (i.e., deep breaths or exercise). The intercostal nerves innervate these muscles.

Figure 1-2

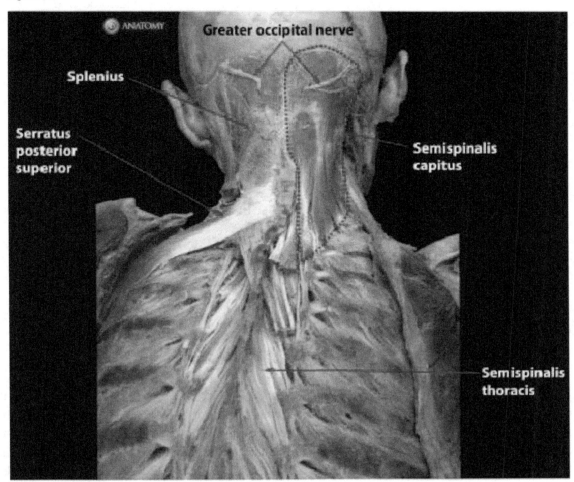

What muscles are responsible for movements of the head?
The neck? The back? How are these muscles innervated?

Intermediate Neck

1   splenius muscle

The **splenius** muscle (**see figure 1-2**) includes a capitus and cervicis
division. Each division works to extend the neck when contracted and is

innervated by dorsal rami. The splenius capitis is located deep to the upper trapezius and rhomboids. It attaches to the spinous processes of C7–T4 and the mastoid process of the skull. The splenius cervicis is more lateral and attaches from spinous processes of T3–T6 to transverse processes of C1–C3.

Deep and Very Deep Muscles of The Back

Deep (erector spinae muscles)

1   iliocostalis

2   longissimus

3   spinalis

Very deep (transversospinalis muscles)

1   semispinalis

2   multifidus

3   rotatores

The **erector spinae** muscle group (**see figure 1-1**) function to extend the back and maintain an erect posture. Innervation is via the dorsal rami. The most lateral muscle is the **iliocostalis**, which attaches from the sacrum to the angle of the ribs. The **longissimus** is located medial to the iliocostalis and has similar attachments. The most medial muscle in this group is the **spinalis**, which attaches to spinous process from the vertebra above and to spinous process from vertebra below. Each muscle can be named for its regional location in the back or neck (e.g., longissimus thoracis, longissimus cervicis).

What muscles are responsible for maintaining alignment of the vertebral column? How are these muscles innervated?

Deep to the erector spinae is the **transversospinalis** muscle group (**see figure 1-2 and 1-3**). Each of the three muscles in this family attach from a spinous process (above) to a transverse process (below). Upon innervation

Figure 1-3

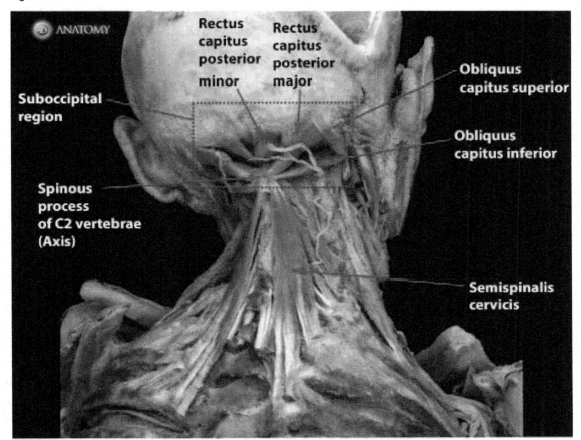

by dorsal rami, these muscles assist in maintaining alignment of the vertebral column (e.g., golf swing). The **semispinalis** spans four to six vertebral segments and is prominent in the cervical region (deep to splenius) and thoracic region. The **greater occipital nerve** (C2) pieces the semispinalis capitus for cutaneous innervation of the posterior skull. (The **multifidus** spans two to four vertebral segments with prominence in the lumbar region. Thirdly, the **rotatores** spans one or two vertebrae and is best observed in the **thoracic** region. Minor muscles of the back include the interspinales (between spinous processes) and levator costorum (transverse process to rib).

The mnemonic device "**3** x **3** x **1** x **3** x **3**" can help identify and group muscles and related anatomy of the back from superficial to deep. Practice writing these down.

1   trapezius, latissimus dorsi, thoracolumbar fascia (3x)

2   rhomboids, levator scapulae, serratus posterior (3x)

3   splenius (1x)

4   iliocostalis, longissimus, spinalis (3x)

5   semispinalis, multifidus, rotatores (3x)

What muscles produce the suboccipital triangle? What are its contents?

The **suboccipital region** and **triangle** are deep to the semispinalis muscle within the inferior, posterior skull region (see figure 1-3). The triangle is formed by three muscular borders. The superior and medial borders are made by **rectus capitis posterior major**. The **rectus capitis posterior minor** is medially located. Together, these muscles assist in extension and lateral rotation of the head and neck. A lateral border joins via the **obliquus capitis superior** and an inferior border by the **obliquus capitis inferior**. These muscles are innervated by the suboccipital nerve (C1), which passes through the middle of the triangle. The **vertebral artery** passes deep to the triangle to supply blood.

See CM 1-2A, 1-2B, 1-2C, and 1-2D for Review.

CM 1-2A

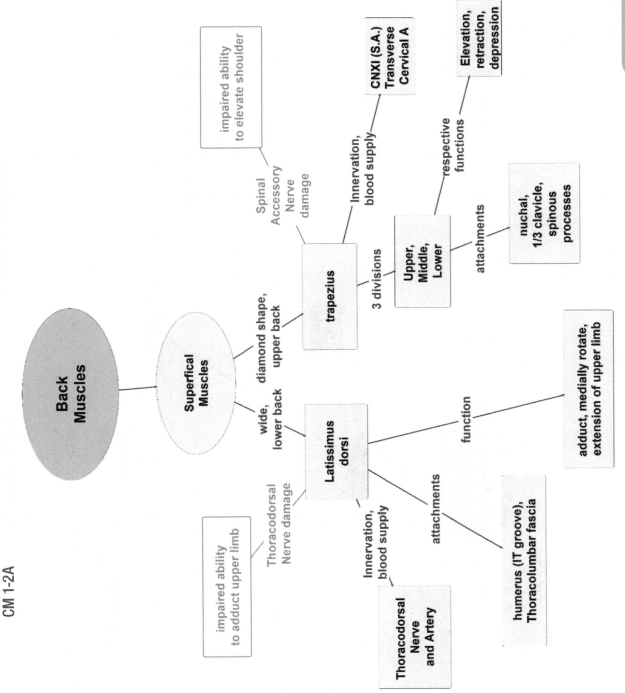

Back Muscles

Superfical Muscles

diamond shape, upper back

wide, lower back

trapezius

Spinal Accessory Nerve damage

impaired ability to elevate shoulder

Innervation, blood supply

CNXI (S.A.) Transverse Cervical A

3 divisions

Upper, Middle, Lower

respective functions

Elevation, retraction, depression

attachments

nuchal, 1/3 clavicle, spinous processes

Latissimus dorsi

Thoracodorsal Nerve damage

impaired ability to adduct upper limb

Innervation, blood supply

Thoracodorsal Nerve and Artery

attachments

humerus (IT groove), Thoracolumbar fascia

function

adduct, medially rotate, extension of upper limb

CM 1-2B

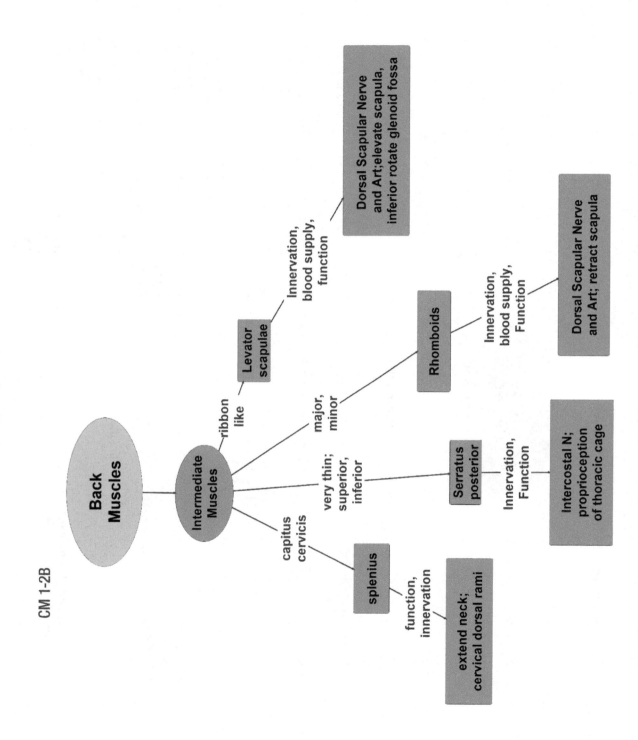

Back Muscles

Intermediate Muscles

ribbon like — Levator scapulae

Innervation, blood supply, function — **Dorsal Scapular Nerve and Art;** elevate scapula, inferior rotate glenoid fossa

major, minor — Rhomboids

Innervation, blood supply, Function — **Dorsal Scapular Nerve and Art;** retract scapula

very thin; superior, inferior — Serratus posterior

Innervation, Function — **Intercostal N;** proprioception of thoracic cage

capitus cervicis — splenius

function, innervation — extend neck; cervical dorsal rami

CM 1-2C

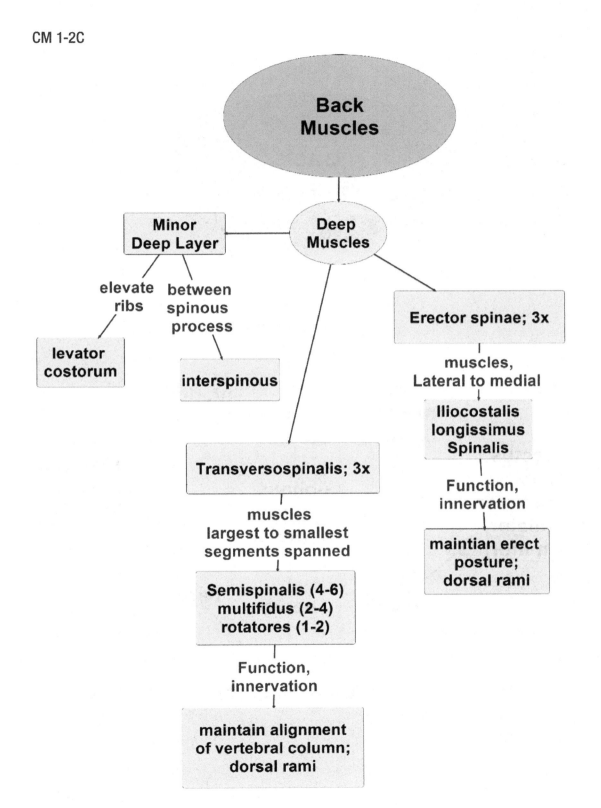

CM 1-2D

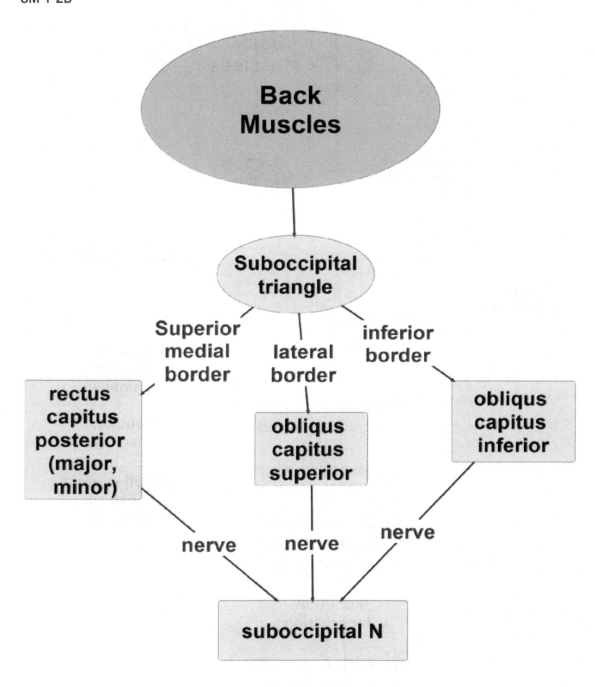

Synthesis Exercise: Create a concept map using items from EXERCISE 1-2A, 1-2B, 1-2C, and 1-2D.

Exercise 1-2A

Primary Category	Secondary Categories	Continuations	Clinical Considerations
Back muscles	Superficial muscles	Trapezius muscle Latissimus dorsi muscle Spinal accessory nerve (CNXI) Transverse cervical artery Elevation Retraction Depression Upper, middle, lower muscle divisions Nuchal line Lateral 1/3 of clavicle Spinous processes Thoracodorsal nerve and artery Adduction, medial rotation of upper limb	Impaired ability to elevate shoulder Impaired ability to adduct upper limb

Exercise 1-2B

Primary Category	Secondary Categories	Continuations
Back muscles	Intermediate muscles	Levator scapulae muscle Rhomboid (major, minor) muscle Serratus posterior muscle Splenius muscle Dorsal scapular nerve and artery Intercostal nerve Proprioception of thoracic cage Extension of neck Dorsal rami

Exercise 1-2C

Primary Category	Secondary Categories	Continuations
Back muscles	Deep muscles	Erector Spinae muscles
		Transversospinalis muscles
		Minor deep layer
		Iliocostalis, Longissimus, Spinalis muscles
		Semispinalis, multifidus, rotatores muscles
		Levator costorum muscle
		Interspinous muscle

Exercise 1-2D

Primary Category	Secondary Categories	Continuations
Back muscles	Suboccipital triangle	Obliquus capitus inferior and superior
		Rectus capitus posterior major and minor
		Suboccipital nerve

III. Spinal Cord and Meninges

Overview of topics for this section:

- Unique features of the spinal cord
- Buffering of the spinal cord
- Spinal meninges
- Severe spinal cord injury
- Spinal cord blood supply
- Great artery of Adamkiewicz
- Cancer metastasis of the spinal cord venous plexus
- Epidural injection
- Lumbar puncture

Does the spinal cord have any unique features? If so, where? What is the cauda equina and where is it located?

The spinal cord has several unique features and landmarks. A **cervical enlargement** occurs from approximately the C4 to the T11 spinal nerves and an inferior **lumbar enlargement** arises from approximately the T11 to the S1 spinal nerves. The spinal cord terminates at the **conus medullaris** at approximately the L2 vertebral level. Remaining spinal nerves extending from the conus medullaris inferiorly are known as the **cauda equina** (~L2 to S2 vertebral level). The **filum terminale** (pial part, at approximately the L2 to S2 vertebral level) is a slender filament of fibrous tissue that continues out of the dural sac; its dural part, from approximately S2, anchors the spinal cord to the coccyx.

What buffers and cushions the spinal cord inside the bony vertebral canal? What 3 layers of spinal meninges surrounds the spinal cord? What is the lumbar cistern and where is it located?

Surroundings and Spinal Meninges of the Spinal Cord

1 vertebral canal
  - epidural fat
2 dura mater
  - no real space; potential space only
3 arachnoid mater
  - subarachnoid space; contains cerebral spinal fluid
4 pia mater

Located between the periosteum of the vertebral canal and the superficial layer of the spinal meninges, the **epidural (extradural) space** is filled with epidural fat to buffer and protect the spinal cord against movements. This space also contains an extensive venous plexus.

The **spinal meninges** is composed of three membrane layers surrounding the spinal cord. The most external layer is the **dura mater** (*tough*

Figure 1-4

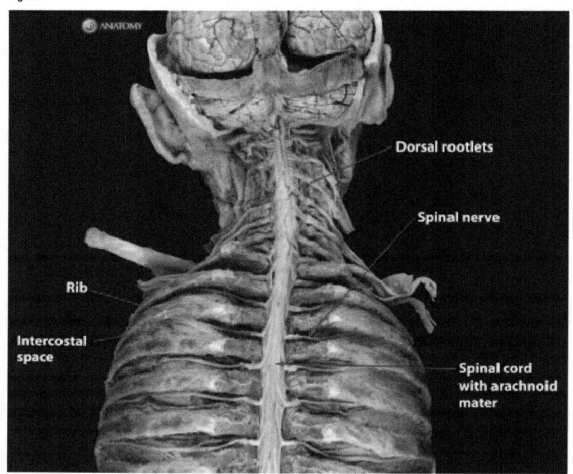

mother), which is relatively tough and protective, is continuous with epineurium of spinal nerves. The dura mater covering the spinal cord is referred to as the **dural sac**, which discontinues at approximately S2. The **arachnoid mater,** which lines the dura mater, is the relatively delicate *spider web like* middle layer of the spinal meninges **(see figure 1-4)**. The **subarachnoid space**, just deep to the arachnoid mater, encloses **cerebral spinal fluid** (CSF). The inner most meningeal layer, called the **pia mater,** is delicate and intimately associated with spinal cord itself. Extensions of the pia mater called denticulate ligaments attach to the arachnoid mater and help suspend the spinal cord.

The cauda equina is located within the **lumbar cistern**. This region is characterized by an increase of subarachnoid space between the conus medullaris (at approximately the L2 vertebral level) and end of the dural sac (at approximately the S2 vertebral level;

At what levels of the spinal cord does severe injury lead to a) a mechanical ventilator; b) normal diaphragm function, but quadriplegia; or c) paraplegia?

The spinal cord can be injured via blunt force trauma (e.g. during an automobile accident or athletic competition). The neuropathology of spinal cord injuries are characterized by three phases: 1) primary injury due to mechanical damage (at time of stimulus); 2) secondary injury (minutes to weeks after stimulus) due to a cascade of biological events, such as inflammation, oxidative stress, and apoptosis; and 3) a chronic phase (days to years after stimulus) that includes demyelination, glial scar tissue, and connective tissue deposition.

The specific level of spinal cord injury determines functional impairments in the patient. For example, injury at C3 vertebral level or above will render the patient unable to initiate normal respiration (phrenic nerve C3, C4, C5) and is quadriplegic (loss of use to all four limbs). These patients consequently require use of a mechanical ventilator. Patients with damage at C6 or below demonstrate normal respiration but quadriplegia. Injuries below T1 include loss of lower limb use or paraplegia.

Where does the spinal cord receive its arterial blood supply? How is venous blood drained from the spinal cord?

The arterial blood supply to the spinal cord itself, is provided primarily by the thoracic aorta and segmental intercostal arteries. The dorsal branch from each intercostal artery supplies a spinal branch to the vertebral body and segmental medullary arteries (anterior, posterior). Blood supply is shared and communicated via two posterior and one anterior spinal arteries, which run the length of the spinal cord. An extensive venous plexus helps drain blood from the spinal cord. This valveless network of veins includes both an internal venous plexus (inside the vertebral canal) and external vertebral plexus (surrounding the vertebral canal).

What is the clinical significance of the great artery of Adamkiewicz?

The great anterior segmental medullary artery of Adamkiewicz is a large supplier of blood to the lower two thirds of the spinal cord. Its origin can vary, but it typically arises from the ninth to the twelfth posterior intercostal artery. Upon damage or obstruction, a patient may experience anterior spinal artery syndrome, which involves loss of urinary function via the bladder, and fecal incontinence. Also, the lower limbs may demonstrate impaired motor function. Surgical correction of an aortic aneurysm risks damage to the great artery of Adamkiewicz.

What contributes to the metastasis of cancer cells through the venous plexus of the vertebral column?

The venous plexus surrounding the spinal cord (or Baston venous plexus) may allow cancer cells from deep pelvic and thoracic veins to metastasize. The spread may include locations such as the vertebral column and brain. The lack of valves in this venous network is considered a mechanism of metastasis.

What is the purpose of an epidural injection? Why should a patient flex the back during this procedure? What layers does the needle tip pass through? Where does the needle stop for this procedure?

Epidural anesthesia can be used to deliver an anesthetic to nerve roots (e.g., for childbirth). This procedure resembles a lumbar puncture, except the needle tip stops in the epidural space, where the anesthetic can then be delivered. Thus, the layers the needle passes through include the skin, subcutaneous fascia, ligamenta flava, and epidural fat.

What is the purpose of a lumbar puncture? What layers does the needle tip pass through and where does the needle stop?

The function of a lumbar puncture is typically to draw cerebrospinal fluid from the spinal cord (e.g., to test for meningitis). The patient assumes a fetal or flexed position to spread the vertebral laminae and spinous processes, and stretch the ligamenta flava between lamina. A local anesthetic is provided to the skin overlying L3/L4 or L4/L5. The needle is introduced to the L3/L4 or L4/L5 level, which reduces risk of injuring the spinal cord because it is inferior to the conus medullaris. The needle tip passes through the skin, subcutaneous fascia, ligamenta flava, epidural fat, and dura and arachnoid mater. Finally, the CSF can be collected within the subarachnoid space.

SEE CM 1-3A, 1-3B, 1-3C, AND 1-3D FOR REVIEW.

CM 1-3A

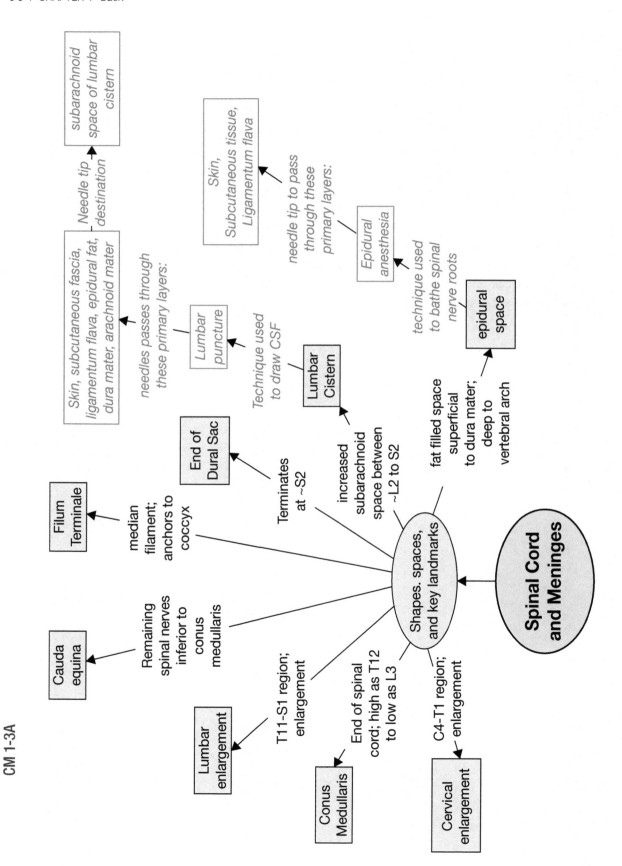

Spinal Cord and Meninges — Shapes, spaces, and key landmarks

- Cervical enlargement — C4-T1 region; enlargement
- Conus Medullaris — End of spinal cord; high as T12 to low as L3
- Lumbar enlargement — T11-S1 region; enlargement
- Cauda equina — Remaining spinal nerves inferior to conus medullaris
- Filum Terminale — median filament; anchors to coccyx
- End of Dural Sac — Terminates at ~S2
- Lumbar Cistern — increased subarachnoid space between ~L2 to S2
  - Lumbar puncture — Technique used to draw CSF
    - Needle tip destination → subarachnoid space of lumbar cistern
    - needles passes through these primary layers: Skin, subcutaneous fascia, ligamentum flava, epidural fat, dura mater, arachnoid mater
- epidural space — fat filled space superficial to dura mater; deep to vertebral arch
  - Epidural anesthesia — technique used to bathe spinal nerve roots
    - needle tip to pass through these primary layers: Skin, Subcutaneous tissue, Ligamentum flava

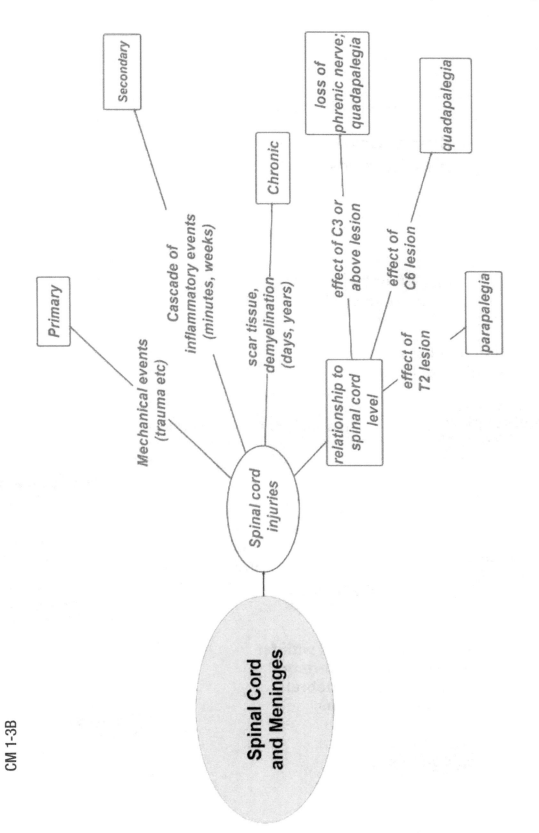

CM 1-3B

CM 1-3C

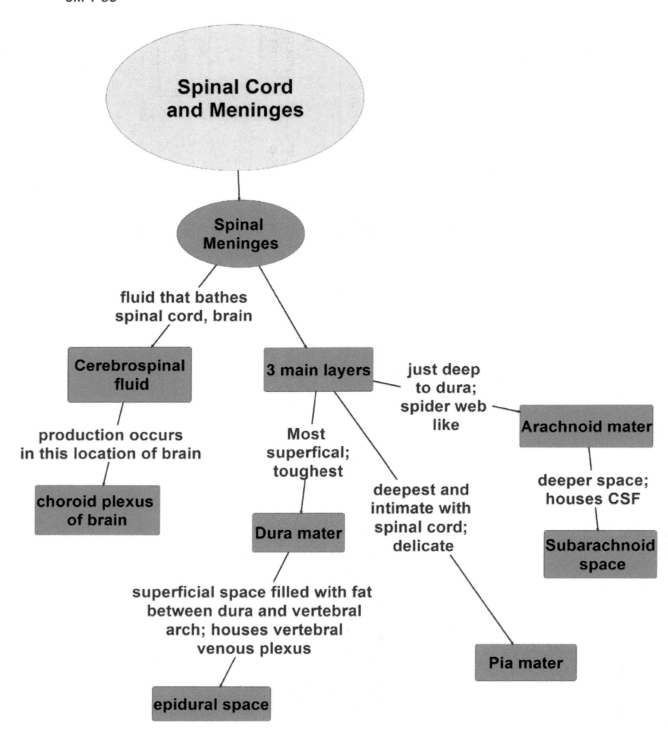

CM 1-3D

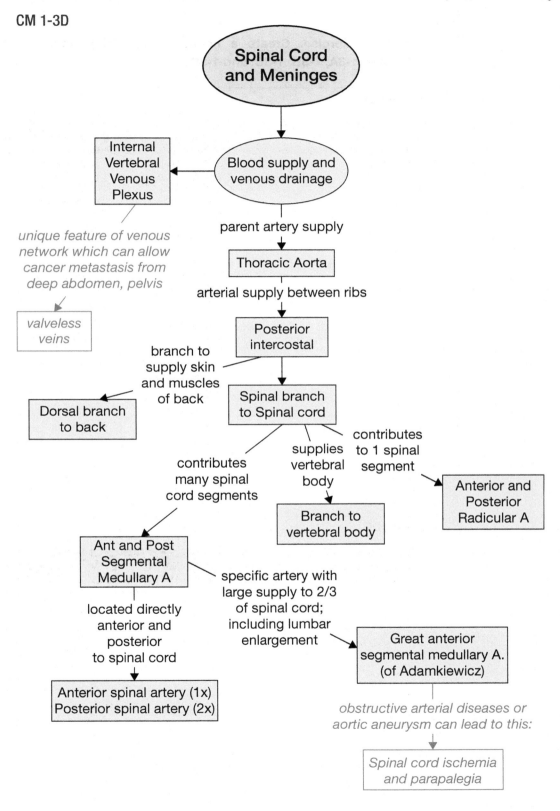

Spinal Cord and Meninges

Blood supply and venous drainage

Internal Vertebral Venous Plexus

unique feature of venous network which can allow cancer metastasis from deep abdomen, pelvis

valveless veins

parent artery supply

Thoracic Aorta

arterial supply between ribs

Posterior intercostal

branch to supply skin and muscles of back

Dorsal branch to back

Spinal branch to Spinal cord

contributes many spinal cord segments

supplies vertebral body

contributes to 1 spinal segment

Branch to vertebral body

Anterior and Posterior Radicular A

Ant and Post Segmental Medullary A

specific artery with large supply to 2/3 of spinal cord; including lumbar enlargement

located directly anterior and posterior to spinal cord

Great anterior segmental medullary A. (of Adamkiewicz)

Anterior spinal artery (1x) Posterior spinal artery (2x)

obstructive arterial diseases or aortic aneurysm can lead to this:

Spinal cord ischemia and parapalegia

Synthesis Exercise: Create a concept map using items from EXERCISE 1-3A, 1-3B, 1-3C, and 1-3D.

Exercise 1-3A

Primary Category	Secondary Categories	Continuations	Clinical Considerations
Spinal Cord and Meninges	Shapes, spaces, and key landmarks	Cervical enlargement	Lumbar puncture
		Conus medullaris	Epidural anesthesia
		Lumbar enlargement	Skin, subcutaneous fascia, ligamentum flava, epidural fat, dura mater, arachnoid mater
		Cauda equina	
		Filum terminale	
		End of dural sac	
		Lumbar cistern	Subarachnoid space of lumbar cistern
		Epidural space	
		3 main layers	Skin, subcutaneous tissue, ligamentum flava, epidural fat
		Cerebrospinal fluid	
		Thoracic aorta	
		Internal vertebral venous plexus	
		C4-T1	
		T12-L3	
		S2	
		L2-S2	
		Anchored at coccyx	

Exercise 1-3B

Primary Category	Primary Clinical Considerations	Secondary Clinical Considerations
Spinal Cord and Meninges	Spinal cord injuries	Mechanical-primary
		Inflammation-secondary
		Scar tissue- chronic
		Spinal cord level injury
		Lesion at C3 or above
		Lesion at C6
		Lesion at T2
		Loss of phrenic nerve
		Quadrapalegia
		Parapalegia

Exercise 1-3C

Primary Category	Secondary Categories	Continuations
Spinal Cord and Meninges	Spinal meninges	3 main layers
		Arachnoid mater
		Pia mater
		Dura mater
		Choroid plexus of the brain
		Subarachnoid space
		Epidural space
		Cerebrospinal fluid

Exercise 1-3D

Primary Category	Secondary Categories	Continuations	Clinical Considerations:
Spinal Cord and Meninges	Shapes, spaces, and key landmarks	Thoracic aorta	Mechanical-primary
		Internal vertebral venous plexus	Inflammation-secondary
		Posterior intercostal artery	Scar tissue- chronic
		Spinal branch to spinal cord	Spinal cord level injury
		Radicular artery	Lesion at C3 or above
		Segmental medullary artery	Lesion at C6
		Spinal artery	Lesion at T2
		Great ant. segmental medullary artery (Adamkiewicz)	Loss of phrenic nerve
			Quadrapalegia
			Parapalegia

IV. Spinal Nerves, Peripheral Nerves, and CN XI

Overview of topics for this section:

- Neuron and nerves
- Spinal versus cranial nerves
- Sensory versus motor nerves
- Segmental versus peripheral nerves
- Somatic versus visceral nerves

What are neurons? What are nerves?

A **neuron** is the basic cell type which communicates electrical messages to, from, and within the central nervous system (CNS). It includes (a) a cell body, which houses the nucleus; (b) dendrites, which extend from the nucleus and receive input; (c) an axon, which relays messages away from the cell body; and (d) an axon terminal, which releases a neurotransmitter. Most sensory neurons are **pseudounipolar**, and motor neurons are typically **multipolar**. Some axons are surrounded by **Schwann cells**, a type of glial cell, which creates a layer of myelination (i.e. *insulation*). The myelin sheath is surrounded by a delicate layer of connective tissue called the **endoneurium**. Taken together, a collection of axons is called a **fascicle**, which is surrounded by connective tissue referred to as the **perineurium**. Fascicles may be grouped together and surrounded by a layer of dense connective tissue called the **epineurium** to create a **nerve**. The blood supply to a nerve is referred to as the **vasa nervorum**.

Spinal versus Cranial Nerves — What is the difference between spinal nerves and cranial nerves? What is unique about CN XI (the spinal accessory nerve)? How many pairs of spinal nerves are present? How are they categorized? What type of neurons are included? How do they exit from the vertebral column?

Each spinal segment gives rise to a right and left spinal nerve, which equals 31 pairs of **spinal nerves**. **Cranial Nerves** (CN; I-XII) exit the skull and include 12 pairs total (I-XII). Unlike the other eleven cranial nerves, CN XI, **the spinal accessory nerve** is unique in that it does not arise from the brain. Instead, it arises from the cervical spinal cord to enter and exit the skull. CN XI innervates the **sternocleidomastoid** and **trapezius** muscles. Spinal nerves are separated into common groups called Cervical (C1-C8), Thoracic (T1-T12), Lumbar (L1-L5), and Sacral (S1-S5). The spinal cord gives rise to dorsal (posterior) and ventral (anterior) rootlets, which immediately fuse to form roots, which carry sensory (dorsal or posterior roots) and motor (ventral or anterior roots) information.

Sensory versus Motor Nerves — What is the difference between a sensory and motor neuron? Do nerves contain both sensory and motor neurons?

Motor neurons exit anteriorly from the spinal cord and transmit efferent electrical impulses to target organs (e.g., skeletal muscle, visceral organs). **Sensory neurons** enter the spinal cord posteriorly and transmit afferent messages to the CNS (e.g., touch, temperature, pain). The distal aspects of the ventral (anterior) and dorsal (posterior) roots fuse to create a short mixed spinal segment and exit laterally from the vertebral column via the intervertebral foramen. Upon exiting the intervertebral foramen, the mixed spinal nerve gives rise to a dorsal (posterior) and ventral (anterior) **ramus**, which can house both sensory and motor neurons. Dorsal (posterior) rami distribute to the posterior neck and back while ventral (anterior) rami course more anteriorly throughout the rest of the body.

Segmental versus Peripheral Nerves — What is a peripheral nerve? What is a nerve plexus? Where are they located? What is an intercostal nerve? How does it differ from a peripheral nerve?

The ventral rami have two main options distally: 1) to remain as an independent spinal nerve (segmental), or 2) fuse with other spinal nerves (**plexus**). The ventral (anterior) rami of spinal nerves T1–T12 are called **intercostal nerves** because of their location between the ribs (i.e., intercostal space). They do not participate in a plexus and remain independent spinal nerves. Thus, distally they are called **segmental nerves**. T1 is an exception to this concept because it participates in the brachial plexus, but is also an intercostal nerve. In contrast to segmental nerves, several ventral (anterior) rami of spinal nerves can fuse to form a plexus within the cervical (C1–C5), brachial (C5–T1), lumbar (L1–L4), and sacral regions (L4–S4). The terminal product of a plexus or integration of spinal nerves is a **peripheral nerve**. For example, the **phrenic nerve**, which innervates the diaphragm, receives contributions from spinal nerves C3, C4, and C5. The **femoral nerve**, which innervates the lower limb, receives contributions from spinal nerves L2, L3, and L4.

What is a dermatome? What is a myotome? How is a dermatome map derived? How is a peripheral nerve map created?

Individual spinal nerves maintain a specific pattern of innervation towards the skin and skeletal muscle. For example, a single spinal nerve conveys afferent (sensory) messages for a specific territory of skin called a **dermatome**. Also, a single spinal nerve supplies efferent (motor) messages to a specific part of skeletal muscle called a **myotome**. A **dermatome map** is derived from patients with proximal spinal nerve lesions. Thus, the resulting territory of skin lacking cutaneous sensation is associated with a dermatome. For example, a patient with a proximal nerve lesion of C6 would likely lose cutaneous sensation over the lateral forearm and hand. Importantly, dermatome patterns may vary within patients (left versus right) and between patients. In contrast to the dermatome map, a **peripheral nerve map** is a pattern of cutaneous innervation collected from patients with a distal lesion to a peripheral nerve. Since a peripheral nerve receives contributions from multiple spinal nerves (i.e. plexus), the cutaneous innervation pattern of a peripheral nerve map is slightly different that of a dermatome map. For example, the lateral cutaneous nerve of the forearm (C5, C6) innervates the lateral forearm, and the radial nerve (C6–C8) innervates the lateral hand.

Somatic versus Visceral Nerves — How are nerves classified based on their destination?

Nerves may be further classified based on their destination. **Somatic nerves** carry messages about skeletal muscle, skin, and joints, and includes both afferent and efferent input. For example, somatic nerves can carry efferent messages to skeletal muscle about contracting (somatic efferent) or afferent messages involving pain of skeletal joints or skin (somatic afferent). Visceral (i.e., splanchnic) nerves carry messages to hollow organs of the thorax, abdomen, and pelvis. This may also include afferent or efferent input. Examples of **visceral nerves** include autonomic nerves to the digestive tract that relay efferent impulses for smooth muscle contractions (visceral efferents) or afferent impulses relaying pain (visceral afferents). Thus, somatic and visceral nerves may contain both sensory (afferent) and/or motor (efferent) neurons.

See CM 1-4A and 1-4B for Review.

CM 1-4A

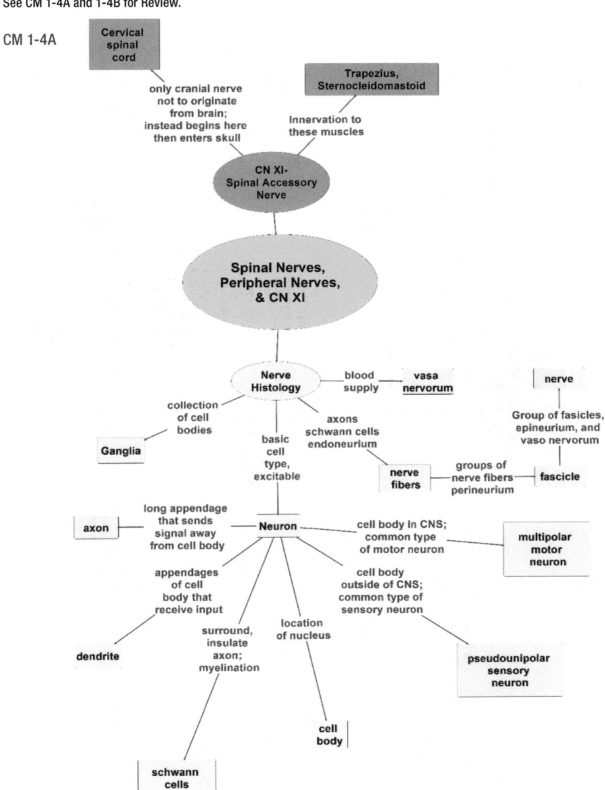

CM 1-4B

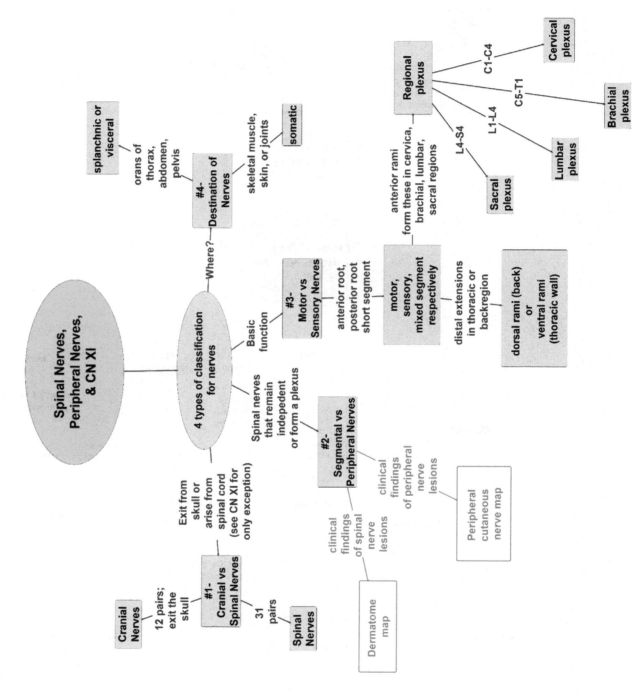

Spinal Nerves, Peripheral Nerves, & CN XI

4 types of classification for nerves

Exit from skull or arise from spinal cord (see CN XI for only exception)

#1- Cranial vs Spinal Nerves

Cranial Nerves

12 pairs; exit the skull

Spinal Nerves

31 pairs

Spinal nerves that remain indepedent or form a plexus

#2- Segmental vs Peripheral Nerves

clinical findings of spinal nerve lesions

Dermatome map

clinical findings of peripheral nerve lesions

Peripheral cutaneous nerve map

Basic function

#3- Motor vs Sensory Nerves

anterior root, posterior root short segment

motor, sensory, mixed segment respectively

anterior rami form these in cervica, brachial, lumbar, sacral regions

distal extensions in thoracic or backregion

dorsal rami (back) or ventral rami (thoracic wall)

Regional plexus

C1-C4 — **Cervical plexus**

C5-T1 — **Brachial plexus**

L1-L4 — **Lumbar plexus**

L4-S4 — **Sacral plexus**

Where?

#4- Destination of Nerves

splanchnic or visceral

orans of thorax, abdomen, pelvis

skeletal muscle, skin, or joints

somatic

Synthesis Exercise: Create a concept map using items from EXERCISE 1-4A and 1-4B.

Exercise 1-4A

Primary Category	Secondary Categories	Continuations
Spinal Nerves, Peripheral Nerves, and CN XI	Nerve histology Spinal accessory nerve (CN XI)	Neuron Ganglia Axon Schwann cells Endoneurium Nerve fiber Dendrite Multipolar neuron Pseudounipolar neuron Fascicle Nerve Cell body typically outside CNS Cell body typically inside CNS Trapezius muscle Sternocleidomastoid muscle Cervical spinal nerve

Exercise 1-4B

Primary Category	Secondary Categories	Continuations	Clinical Considerations
Spinal Nerves, Peripheral Nerves, and CN XI	4 types of classification for nerves	Cranial vs spinal nerves Segmental vs peripheral nerves otor vs sensory nerves Destination of nerves 12 pairs exit skull 31 pairs derived from spinal cord Anterior root Posterior root Mixed spinal segment Anterior (ventral) rami Posteror (dorsal) rami Somatic nerves	Dermatome map Peripheral cutaneous nerve map

Primary Category	Secondary Categories	Continuations	Clinical Considerations
		Splanchnic (visceral) nerves	
		Skeletal muscle	
		Joints	
		Skin	
		Hollow organs	
		Cervical plexus	
		Brachial plexus	
		Lumbar plexus	
		Sacral plexus	
		C1-C4	
		C5-T1	
		L1-L4	
		L4-S4	

Image Credits

- Fig. 1-1: Copyright © 2016 by 4D Anatomy. Reprinted with permission.
- Fig. 1-2: Copyright © 2016 by 4D Anatomy. Reprinted with permission.
- Fig. 1-3: Copyright © 2016 by 4D Anatomy. Reprinted with permission.
- Fig. 1-4: Copyright © 2016 by 4D Anatomy. Reprinted with permission.

CHAPTER 2
Lower Limb

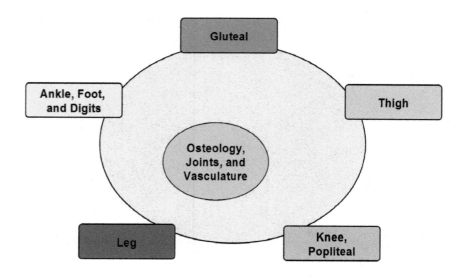

Brief Introduction

What are the basic regions of the lower limb? Consider the gluteal, thigh, knee, leg, ankle, dorsal foot, plantar foot, and digits.

The **gluteal** region (i.e., buttocks) is a posterior transition site from the pelvis to the lower limb. Just inferior to this is the **thigh,** which houses a single bone (femur) and several large muscles for extension, flexion, and adduction. The **knee joint** is an articulation site between bones of the thigh and leg. Located on the posterior aspect of the knee is the **popliteal region** that houses important neurovasculature. The **leg** contains 2 bones: the tibia (medial) and fibula (lateral). Several muscles of the leg help plantar flex (i.e., stand on toes) and dorsiflex (i.e., point toes superiorly) the foot. Inversion (medial angling) and eversion (lateral angling) of the foot also takes place via muscles located in the leg. The **ankle joint** articulates bones of the leg with the **talus** (ankle bone). In the anatomical position, the foot has a dorsal surface (superior) and a plantar surface (inferior). **Digits (1–5)** extend directly from the bones of the foot.

I. Osteology, Joints, and Vasculature

Overview of key topics for this section:

- Ball and socket joint of the hip
- Femoral ligaments
- Femoral bone fractures
- Angle of inclination
- Hip replacement
- Knee joint ligaments
- Bursitis of the knee
- Unhappy triad
- Arches of the foot and fallen arch
- Vasculature to the lower limb
- Lymphedema
- Muscle pump

The hip is a ball and socket joint and includes a wide range of motion. What underlying osteology is responsible for this?

The hip. The **acetabulum**, composed of three types of **pelvic bone** (**pubic**, **ilium**, **ischium**), forms the hollow socket of the hip that accepts the femoral head. The inferior aspect of the acetabulum is not completely closed by bone. Rather, the **transverse acetabular ligament** spans this region and completes the circular shape of the acetabulum). A C-shaped area composed of articular membrane (the **lunate surface**) is also present on the medial aspect of the acetabulum and reduces friction in the hip joint. Ball and socket joints, like the hip, promote a wide range of motion including extension, flexion, medial and lateral rotation, abduction, adduction, and circumduction. An extension of the femoral head is the **ligament to the head of the femur**. This ligament houses an arterial branch, the **acetabular branch of the obturator artery,** which helps supply the femoral head. This ligament attaches to the center of the acetabulum (its **fovea**), which is not covered by articular membrane. Three femoral ligaments help further stabilize the hip joint by limiting excessive movements. The **iliofemoral ligament,** located superiorly, is shaped like a *Y*. It functions to resist hyperextension at the hip. The **pubofemoral ligament,** located inferiorly, prevents over abduction at the hip. The third ligament, the **ischiofemoral ligament**, is located on the posterior aspect.

What is a fractured hip? A dislocated hip? A hip replacement?

A **hip fracture** may occur in the proximal end of the femur at the femoral head, femoral neck, intertrochanteric crest, or subtrochanteric. Debilitating falls in the elderly is a common cause for hip fractures due to bone and muscle weakness (osteoporosis and sarcopenia, respectively). Also, trauma to the hip during a car accident or athletic competition is associated with proximal femoral fracturing.

A **dislocated hip** results from subluxation (i.e., removal, or exit) of the femoral head from the acetabulum. This injury can occur following the introduction of excessive force driven superiorly through the femur. It may also increase the risk of damage to the arterial supply to the femoral head and neck, such as the circumflex femoral arteries, and can result in avascular necrosis if undetected.

Osteoarthritis is a risk factor for requiring a **hip replacement**. Chronic wear and tear of the articular membrane within the hip joint can cause daily discomfort in patients while standing or walking. If conservative treatments are ineffective, a complete replacement of the femoral head with a prosthesis may be required.

What is the main source of structural support for the thigh? The lower leg? What unique bony features help translate movements in these regions?

The thigh. The femur bone provides structural support for the thigh. The **femoral head** articulates with the acetabulum of the pelvis and the **femoral neck** attaches the head to the femoral shaft. On the femoral shaft, two protuberances serve as sites of muscle attachment: the greater and lesser trochanter. The **greater trochanter** is larger and located on the superior and proximal aspects of the shaft. The **lesser trochanter** is smaller and located posteriorly on the shaft. An intertrochanteric line (anterior) and crest (posterior) connect the greater and lesser trochanter. The **gluteal tuberosity** is a site of attachment for the gluteus maximus muscle on the proximal femoral shaft. A ridge located posteriorly called the **linea aspera** is another site of muscle attachment. It is a continuation of the supracondylar line from the distal femur. The **medial and lateral epicondyles** are distal expansions of the femoral ends. Vertical fibers of the adductor magnus muscle attach to the medial epicondyle at the **adductor tubercle**. **Medial and lateral condyles** of the femur are rounded in shape and articulate with the tibial plateau to create the knee joint. Key landmarks of surface anatomy for the thigh region include the greater trochanter (8–10 cm below the iliac crest), the medial and lateral epicondyles near the knee, and the patella (knee cap).

The knee joint and leg. The **tibia** (medial) and **fibula** (lateral) bones provide structural support for the leg region. The **tibial plateau**, including the **medial and lateral tibial condyles**, accepts the femoral condyles to create the knee joint. Primary movements of the knee are extension and flexion. Several key ligaments are bound between the femur, tibia, and the fibula to maintain the structural integrity of the knee joint. The **anterior and posterior cruciate ligaments** (ACL and PCL, respectively) are centrally located in the knee and cross one another. The ACL is a band of fibrous cartilage which runs from the superior and lateral aspect of the femur to the inferior and medial aspect of tibia. It prevents excessive anterior translation of the tibia relative to the femur. Similarly, the PCL attaches from the superior and medial aspect of the femur to the inferior and medial aspect of the tibia. It prevents excessive posterior translation of the tibia relative to the femur. A small, superior space between the medial and lateral tibial condyles is called the **intercondylar area** and serves as an attachment site for the cruciate ligaments. The **collateral ligaments** help prevent excessive medial and lateral movements. For example, the **medial collateral ligament** (MCL), or **tibial collateral ligament** (TCL), is located medially on the knee joint and prevents medial movements. In contrast, the **lateral collateral ligament** (LCL), or **fibular collateral ligament** (FCL), is found laterally and prevents lateral movements. The articulation of the femur and tibia is buffered by 2 separate menisci: the medial (C-shaped) and lateral **menisci** (nearly circular in shape). These fibrocartilage structures are specifically located between the condyles of the femur and the tibial plateau. The MCL and medial meniscus form an attachment to one another, but the LCL and lateral meniscus do not share an attachment. Thus, tearing of the MCL often leads to disruption of the medial meniscus.

Furthermore, **Gerdy's tubercle** (anterolateral) is a site of attachment for the **iliotibial** (IT) band on the proximal tibia. The **tibial tuberosity** is located anteriorly on the proximal tibia and serves as an attachment site for the **patellar tendon**. On the posterior tibial shaft is a **soleal line,** whereby the **soleus muscle** attaches. Distally, the **medial malleolus** of the tibia is a distal expansion which helps create the ankle joint. On the lateral aspect of the leg is the fibula. The fibular head articulates with the proximal tibia and the fibular neck connects the head and shaft. A **lateral malleolus** is found distally on the fibula and helps reinforce the ankle joint. Taken together, the distal tibia and fibula creates an up-side down U-like to accept the **talus** (ankle bone). An **interosseous membrane** helps stabilize the tibia and fibular together. Key landmarks of surface anatomy for the leg region include the fibular head, anterior border of the tibial shaft, and the medial and lateral malleoli for the ankle joint.

What is the angle of inclination?

The angle between the shaft and neck of the femur can vary among individuals. A common angle occurs between 120 and 135 degrees. However, if the angle is < 120 degrees, it is called **coxa vara**. If the angle is > 135 degrees, it is called **coxa valga**. Also, the angle of inclination typically decreases with aging.

What is the anterior and posterior drawer test of the knee?

An initial clinical determination for a torn ACL or PCL is accomplished by the drawer test. During the test, the patient is supine with the hip flexed (45 degrees) and knee flexed (90 degrees). The **anterior draw test** involves pulling the tibia anteriorly. A non-injured ACL prevents excessive anterior translation of the tibia relative to the femur. The test indicates that the ACL is torn when the tibia translates anterior more than a normal or uninjured knee. The **posterior drawer test** is similar, but pushes the tibia in a posterior direction. This test evaluates whether the PCL has been torn.

What is an unhappy triad of the knee?

Due to excessive abduction and lateral rotation of the leg during a fixed stance (planted), the ACL, MCL, and medial meniscus can be torn simultaneously (the medial meniscus may tear completely or partially). This injury is called an unhappy triad and typically occurs in athletic competition (e.g., a football tackle).

What bones account for both structural support and dynamic movement of the distal lower limb (i.e. ankle, foot, and digits)?

Ankle and hindfoot. The distal tibia (medial malleolus) and distal fibula (lateral malleolus) create a rectangular socket that accepts the **talus bone**, creating the ankle joint. Its primary functions include dorsiflexion (digits and foot angled superiorly), plantarflexion (digits and foot angled inferiorly), eversion (foot angled laterally), and inversion (foot angled medially). The **calcaneus bone** (i.e. heel bone) resides just inferior to the talus bone and is susceptible to fracture when excessive force is driven superiorly through this bone (e.g., landing from parachuting). Together, the talus and calcaneus make up the hindfoot. Joints in this region are typically named for the bones that articulate (e.g., talocalcaneonavicular, subtalar).

    Midfoot. The **navicular** (anterior-medial) and **cuboid** (anterior-lateral) bones articulate with the talus and calcaneus bones, respectively. Medial, middle, and lateral **cuneiform** bones are similar to carpal bones of the wrist which articulate with the metatarsal bones of the forefoot. Joints in this region are also typically named for the bones that articulate (e.g., calcaneocuboid, tarsometatarsal)

Forefoot. Metatarsal bones (numbered 1–5 from medial to lateral) are similar to the metacarpal bones of the hand. The **phalanges** attach distally to the metatarsal bones. The first digit has only two phalanges, whereas digits 2-5 have three phalanges each. Likeother regions, joints in the forefoot are typically named for the bones that articulate (e.g., metatarsophalangeal, interphalangeal)

Ligaments. Ligaments create stability and typically their names reflect their bony attachment sites. On the medial aspect of the ankle is the **deltoid group** including the (1) **anterior tibiotalar**, (2) **tibionavicular**, (3) **tibiocalcaneal**, and (4) **posterior tibiotalar** ligaments. These ligaments help prevent excessive eversion (or lateral angling) of the ankle joint. Ligaments on the lateral ankle prevent excessive inversion (or medial angling) of the ankle joint and include the (1) **anterior tibiofibular**, (2) **posterior tibiofibular**, (3) **anterior talofibular**, (4) **calcaneofibular**, (5) **posterior talofibular**, and (6) **superior and posterior fibular retinaculum**. On the medial and plantar aspect of the foot is the plantar **calcaneonavicular ligament** (spring ligament), which helps maintain the medial longitudinal arch of the foot by connecting the calcaneus and navicular bones. The long and short **plantar ligaments** connect the calcaneus and cuboid bones. On the anterior aspect of the ankle joint are the superior and inferior **extensor retinacula,** which help prevent bow stringing of the extensor tendons in this region. Furthermore, three arches of the foot (medial, longitudinal, and transverse) also provide structural support and promote force distribution through the foot during the stance phase of gait. Support for the aches consist of muscles (**tibialis** anterior, tibialis posterior, **flexor hallucis longus, flexor digitorum longus, plantar muscles**), the **plantar aponeurosis**, plantar ligaments, and the spring ligament.

What arteries supply the lower limb?

Gluteal. Branching from the **internal iliac artery**, the superior and inferior **gluteal arteries** constitute the major arterial blood supply to the gluteal region. The superior gluteal artery courses above the **piriformis muscle** to supply the **gluteus medius**, **gluteus minimus**, **gluteus maximus**, and **tensor fasciae latae muscles**. The inferior gluteal artery exits below the piriformis muscle to supply the gluteus maximus, piriformis, and **quadratus femoris muscles**.

Thigh and Hip Joint. The **external iliac artery** continues as the **femoral artery** as it passes under the **inguinal ligament** to enter the thigh.

The deep artery to the thigh (**profunda femoris**) quickly branches from the femoral artery to supply the majority of thigh muscles. It also gives rise to the medial and lateral **circumflex femoral arteries**, which supply the femoral head and neck. The artery to the head of the femur courses inside of the ligament of the head of the femur. It branches from the **obturator artery** to supply the proximal head of the femur, but experiences reduced blood flow once the bone stops growing (around 15 years of age). The femoral artery continues distally through the adductor canal of the thigh.

Knee joint and leg. The femoral artery gives rise to the **popliteal artery** as it passes through the adductor hiatus of the adductor magnus muscle. Within the popliteal region, the popliteal artery gives rise to five **genicular branches** that supply the knee joint: (1) superior medial, (2) superior lateral, (3) inferior medial, (4) inferior lateral, and (5) middle genicular arteries. Several **anastomoses** occur amongst these arteries. The leg receives arterial blood from anterior and posterior **tibial arteries** which bifurcate from the popliteal artery. The anterior tibial artery pierces through the interosseous membrane of the leg to supply the anterior **compartment muscles,** and the posterior tibial artery supplies the posterior compartment muscles.

Ankle joint, foot, digits. The anterior tibial artery courses through the anterior compartment of the leg and gives rise to the **dorsalis pedis artery** on the dorsal surface of the foot. The **lateral tarsal** and **dorsalis pedis** arteries contribute to the **arcuate arch** in this region. Extending from this **arterial arch** is the **metatarsal arteries** and **dorsal digital arteries**. Main supply to the plantar surface of the foot occurs via the posterior tibial artery which bifurcates into the medial and lateral **plantar arteries**. These arteries supply the medial and lateral aspects of the plantar surface of the foot, respectively. Also, a calcaneal branch arises from the posterior tibial artery to supply the heel of the foot. Distally, the lateral plantar artery gives rise to the **deep plantar arch**. This arch produces the **plantar metatarsal arteries** and **plantar digital arteries** for supply to the digits.

What drains venous blood from the lower limb? What is the muscle pump?

Superficial venous drainage of the lower limb occurs via the **great saphenous** and **small saphenous veins**. The distal aspect of the great saphenous vein resides over the dorsum of the foot and courses over the medial aspect of the lower limb. It passes through the **saphenous opening** of the fascia lata to meet the **femoral vein**. Similarly, the small saphenous vein courses over the dorsum of the foot and enters the popliteal space. It then meets the **popliteal vein**. Several other deeper veins course along with the arteries of the lower limb, such as the deep vein of the thigh (**profunda femoris vein**), anterior and posterior **tibial veins**, and **plantar** and **dorsal veins** of the foot. Together, venous valves and skeletal muscle contractions (the **muscle pump**) of the lower limb help return venous blood proximally to pelvis region.

How is lymph fluid drained from the lower limb? What is lymphedema? What causes elephantiasis?

Lymphatic drainage of the lower limb occurs superficially and deep through **lymphatic vessels**. This extracellular fluid may pass through **popliteal lymph nodes** of the posterior knee and **inguinal lymph nodes** (superficial, deep) surrounding the saphenous opening before entering the **iliac lymph nodes**. **Lymphedema** occurs when lymph fluid is blocked from normal return and causes **edema** (swelling) of the lower limb. **Elephantiasis tropica** is a type of lymphedema caused by the roundworm, filariasis. Clinical trials have demonstrated that antibiotics may be an effective therapeutic against this condition.

See CM 2-1A, 2-1B, 2-2A, 2-2B, 2-2C, and 2-3A for Review.

CM 2-1A

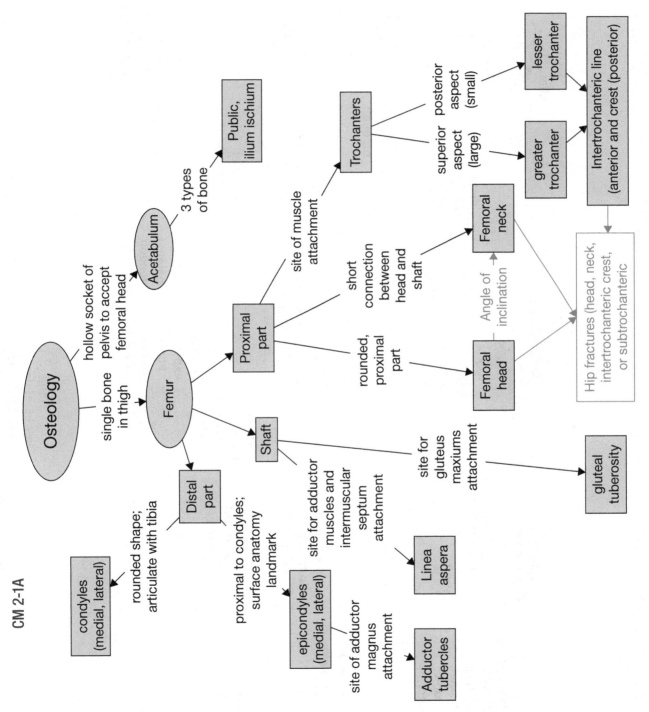

CHAPTER 2

CM 2-1B

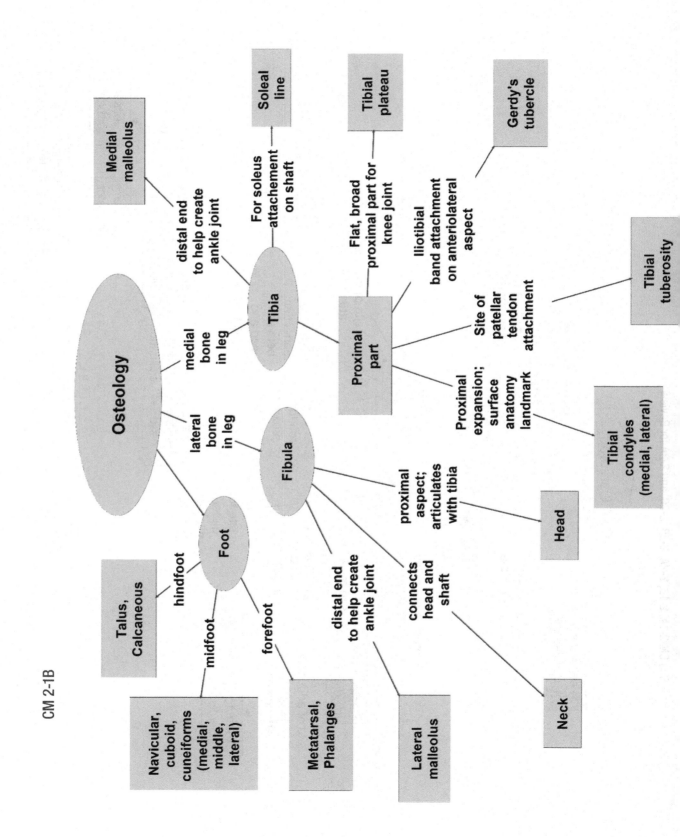

CHAPTER 2

CM 2-2A

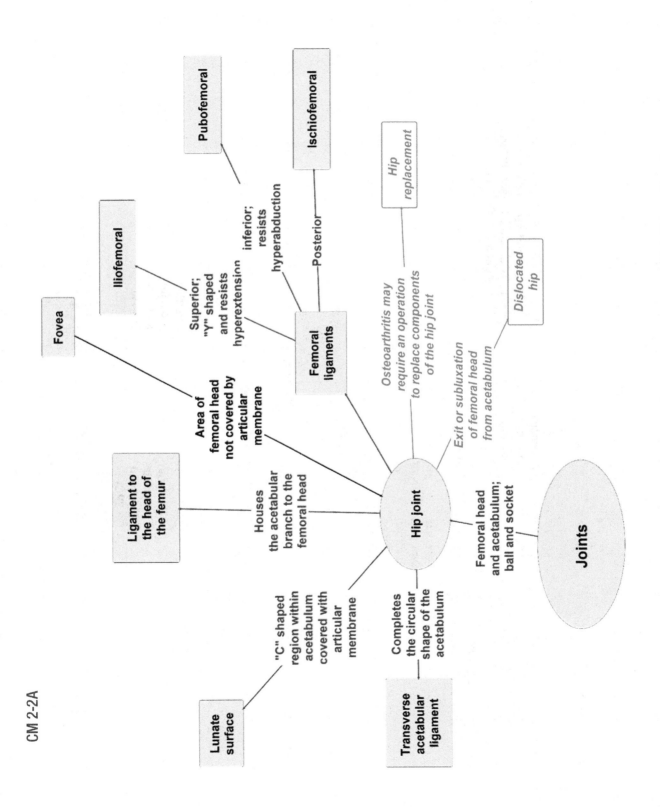

Pubofemoral

Ischiofemoral

Hip replacement

Iliofemoral

inferior; resists hyperabduction

Posterior

Fovea

Superior; "Y" shaped and resists hyperextension

Dislocated hip

Area of femoral head not covered by articular membrane

Femoral ligaments

Osteoarthritis may require an operation to replace components of the hip joint

Ligament to the head of the femur

Houses the acetabular branch to the femoral head

Exit or subluxation of femoral head from acetabulum

Hip joint

Femoral head and acetabulum; ball and socket

Lunate surface

"C" shaped region within acetabulum covered with articular membrane

Completes the circular shape of the acetabulum

Transverse acetabular ligament

Joints

CM 2-2B

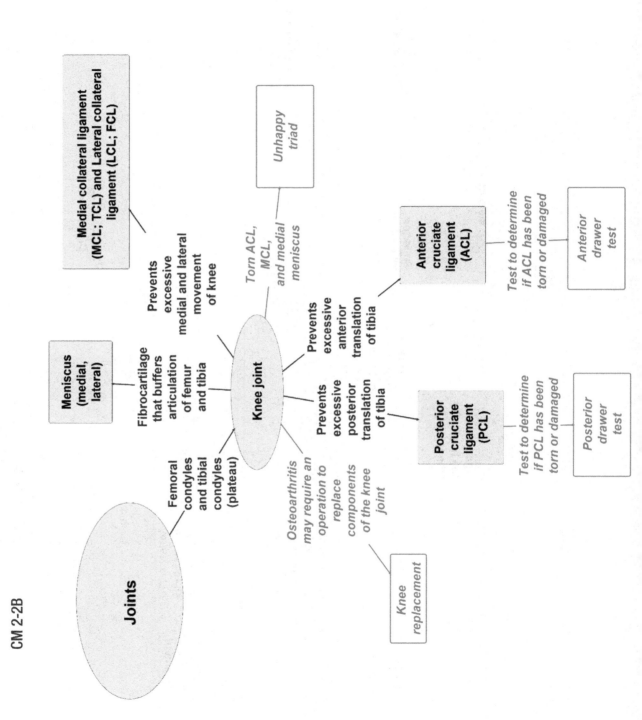

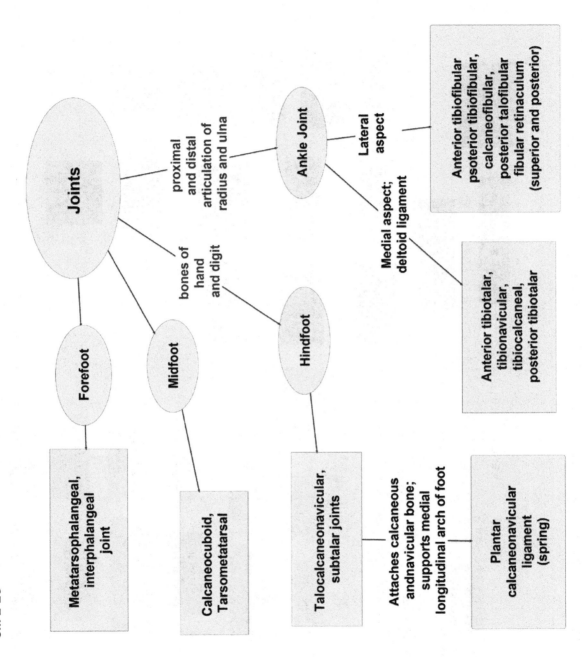

CM 2-2C

Joints

proximal and distal articulation of radius and ulna

Ankle Joint

Lateral aspect

Anterior tibiofibular, psoterior tibiofibular, calcaneofibular, posterior talofibular, fibular retinaculum (superior and posterior)

Medial aspect; deltoid ligament

Anterior tibiotalar, tibionavicular, tibiocalcaneal, posterior tibiotalar

bones of hand and digit

Hindfoot

Talocalcaneonavicular, subtalar joints

Attaches calcaneous andnavicular bone; supports medial longitudinal arch of foot

Plantar calcaneonavicular ligament (spring)

Forefoot

Metatarsophalangeal, interphalangeal joint

Midfoot

Calcaneocuboid, Tarsometatarsal

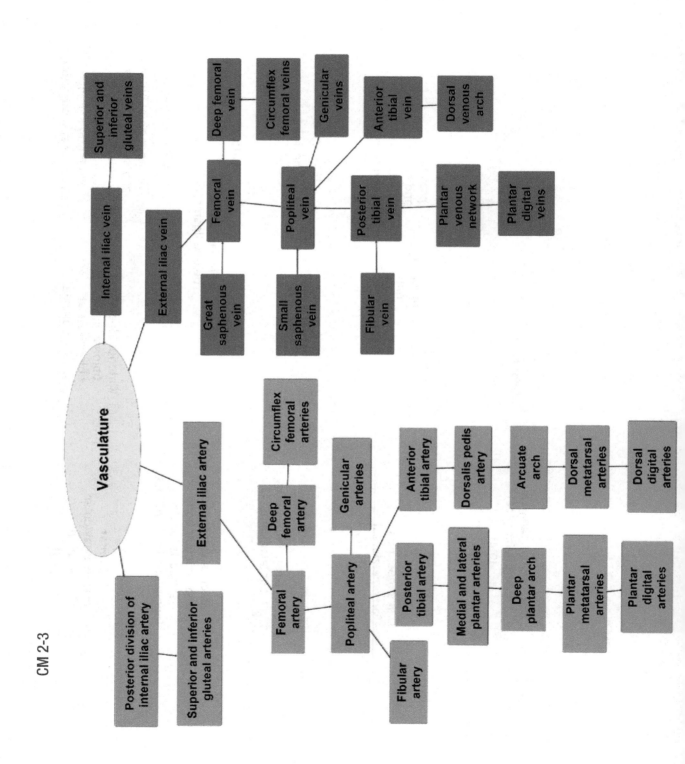

CM 2-3

Synthesis Exercise: Create a concept map using items from EXERCISE 2-1A, 2-1B, 2-2A, 2-2B, 2-2C, and 2-3A.

Exercise 2-1A

Primary Category	Secondary Categories	Continuations	Clinical Considerations
Osteology	Acetabulum	Pubic, ilium, ischium	Hip fractures
	Femur	Proximal femur	Angle of inclination
		Femoral shaft	
		Distal femur	
		Femoral head	
		Femoral neck	
		Trochanters	
		Greater trochanter	
		Lesser trochanter	
		Intertrochanteric line and crest	
		Gluteal tuberosity	
		Linea Aspera	
		Femoral epicondyles	
		Femoral condyles	

Exercise 2-1B

Primary Category	Secondary Categories	Continuations
Osteology	Tibia	Proximal tibia
	Fibula	Medial malleolus
	Foot	Soleal line
		Fibular head
		Fibular neck
		Lateral malleolus
		Metatarsal
		Phalanges
		Navicular
		Cuboid
		Cuneiforms (medial, middle, lateral)
		Talus
		Calcaneous

Exercise 2-2A

Primary Category	Secondary Categories	Continuations	Clinical Considerations
Joints	Hip joint	Femoral ligaments	Hip replacement
		Ligament to the head of the femur	Dislocated hip
		Fovea	
		Lunate surface	
		Transverse acetabular ligament	
		Iliofemoral	
		Pubofemoral	
		Ischiofemoral	

Exercise 2-2B

Primary Category	Secondary Categories	Continuations	Clinical Considerations
Joints	Knee joint	Mediscus (medial, lateral)	Unhappy triad
		Medial collateral ligament	Anterior drawer test
		Lateral collateral ligament	Posterior drawer test
		Anterior cruciate ligament	Knee replacement
		Posterior cruciate ligament	

Exercise 2-2C

Primary Category	Secondary Categories	Continuations
Joints	Ankle joint	Anterior tibiofibular lig.
	Hindfoot	Posterior tibiofibular lig.
	Midfoot	Calcaneofibular lig.
	Forefoot	Posterior talofibular lig.
		Fibular retinaculum ligament (superior and posterior)
		Anterior tibiotalar lig.
		Tibionavicular lig.
		Tibiocalcaneal lig.
		Posterior tibiotalar lig.
		Talocalcaneonavicular joint

Primary Category	Secondary Categories	Continuations
		Subtalar joint
		Calcaneocuboid joint
		Tarsometatarsal joint
		Metatarsophalangeal joint
		Interphalangeal joint

Exercise 2-3

Primary Category	Arterial	Venous
Vasculature	Posterior division of internal iliac artery	Internal iliac vein
	Superior and inferior gluteal arteries	Superior and inferior gluteal veins
	External iliac artery	External iliac vein
	Femoral artery	Femoral vein
	Deep femoral artery	Deep femoral vein
	Circumflex femoral arteries	Circumflex femoral veins
	Popliteal artery	Popliteal vein
	Genicular arteries	Genicular veins
	Fibular artery	Fibular vein
	Posterior tibial artery	Posterior tibial vein
	Anterior tibial artery	Anterior tibial vein
	Medial and lateral plantar arteries	Plantar venous network
	Deep plantar arch	Plantar digital veins
	Plantar metatarsal arteries	Dorsal venous arch
	Plantar digital arteries	
	Dorsalis pedis artery	
	Arcuate Arch	
	Dorsal metatarsal arteries	
	Dorsal digital arteries	

II. Gluteal

Overview of key topics for this section:

- Gluteal muscles (large, small) and actions
- Neurovasculature of this region
- Cutaneous innervation
- Trendelenburg testing, sign, and gait
- Gluteal intramuscular injections
- Piriformis syndrome

What are the large gluteal muscles What are their functions? What comprises their neurovasculature?

Large Gluteal Muscles

1 gluteus maximus
2 gluteus medius
3 gluteus minimus

Three large gluteal muscles are named for relative size. The largest is the **gluteus maximus**, a powerful extensor of the hip starting from a flexed position (e.g., sitting to standing up). It attaches primarily to the lateral sacrum and iliotibial tract (band); some fibers attach to the gluteal tuberosity. Its innervation includes the inferior gluteal nerve (L5-S2) and blood supply occurs via both the superior and inferior gluteal artery.

The medium sized **gluteus medius** is deep to the gluteus maximus **(see figure 2-1).** It helps abduct the lower limb at the hip and maintain a horizontal pelvis during the transfer of weight (e.g., walking). The superior gluteal nerve (L4–S1) innervates the gluteus medius and the superior gluteal artery supplies blood. The smaller sized **gluteus minimus** resides under the gluteus medius, which attaches to the central ilium and the greater trochanter of the femur. It shares similar actions, innervation, and blood supply as the gluteus medius.

Figure 2-1

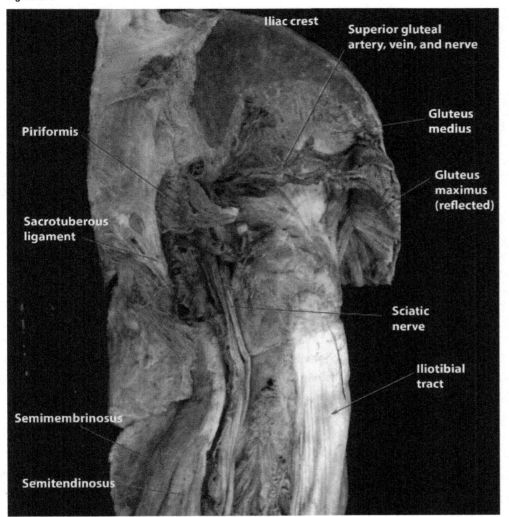

Iliac crest

Superior gluteal
artery, vein, and nerve

Piriformis

Gluteus
medius

Gluteus
maximus
(reflected)

Sacrotuberous
ligament

Sciatic
nerve

Iliotibial
tract

Semimembrinosus

Semitendinosus

What are the small gluteal muscles? What are their
functions? What comprises their neurovasculature?

Small Gluteal Muscles

1   piriformis
2   superior gemellus

3   obturator internus

4   inferior gemellus

5   quadratus femoris

Several smaller muscles reside deep to the gluteus maximus. The pear-shaped **piriformis muscle** serves as a good landmark for identification of surrounding structures in this region. Major gluteal nerves and arteries typically exit just above and below the piriformis muscle. It attaches to the lateral sacrum and the greater trochanter, it is innervated by S1–S2, and it can laterally rotate the lower limb. Just inferior to the piriformis, are the **superior and inferior gemelli** muscles, which attach from the **ischial spine** to the greater trochanter. They also function as lateral rotators. Innervation of the superior gemallus is via the nerve to the obturator internus (see below) and innervation of the inferior gemallus is via the nerve to the quadratus femoris (see below). The **obturator internus** muscle, which also participates in lateral rotation of the lower limb, lies between the two gemelli muscles. It extends from the medial aspect of the obturator membrane through the lesser sciatic foramen and attaches distally to the greater trochanter. The most inferiorly located muscle in this category, the **quadratus femoris**, attaches from the ischial tuberosity to the intertrochanteric crest of the femur. Innervation is via the **nerve to the quadratus femoris**. All of these lateral rotator muscles (gemelli, obturator internus, and quatratus femoris) receive blood via the inferior gluteal artery. The **sciatic nerve** is the largest nerve in humans and originates from the anterior rami of L4–S1. It courses just below the piriformis muscle and is destined for the lower limb as the tibia and fibular nerve. The **posterior cutaneous nerve of the thigh** (S1–S3) runs on the medial aspect of the sciatic nerve and provides cutaneous sensation on the posterior thigh. Cutaneous sensation over the gluteal region occurs via the **clunial nerves,** which include the (1) **superior clunial** (central gluteal), (2) **medial clunial** (near midline gluteal), and (3) **inferior clunial** (near the gluteal fold).

What is the Trendelenburg test?

The **Trendelenburg test** is used to determine the functionality of the gluteus medius muscle. For example, a patient is instructed to stand on one foot only. During a negative Trendelenburg test, the pelvis will remain level or horizontal due to contraction of the gluteus medius muscle on the ipsilateral side. If the superior gluteal nerve is damaged (i.e., pelvic trauma), the pelvis shifts inferiorly to the contralateral side when weight is placed on the side of injury. The pelvis does not appear level or horizontal, which indicates of a positive **Trendelenburg sign**. A **Trendelenburg gait** occurs when a patient with damage to the superior gluteal nerve attempts a walking gait and demonstrates a swinging gait or waddle due to the uneven shift of the pelvis.

Where is a safe location for an intramuscular injection of the gluteal region?

A safe and effective **intramuscular injection** to the gluteal region e.g., steroids or vaccination) should occur in the upper, lateral quadrant. This approach typically prevents damage to the neurovasculature in the gluteal region which arises medially, , such as superior gluteal artery and nerve. To perform an intramuscular injection, the clinician places the index finger on the anterior superior iliac spine (ASIS) with digit 1 (thumb) angled anteriorly and inferiorly. The needle tip is inserted between the index and middle fingers for safety.

What is sciatica?

Compression or irritation to sciatic nerves may frequently cause numbness or paresthesia (a pins and needles sensation) down the lower limb of the affected side. It can be caused by a variety of factors including extensive sitting, hypertrophy of the piriformis muscle, and sitting on a large wallet (wallet sciatica). An intervertebral disc herniation can produce similar symptoms.

What is piriformis syndrome?

The location and course of the sciatic nerve may vary during development. If the sciatic nerve passes directly through or above the piriformis muscle, the patient may experience sciatica-like symptoms due to compression of the sciatic nerve. Abnormal hypertrophy of the piriformis muscle can also have similar effects. This condition is known as **piriformis syndrome**.

See CM 2-4A for Review.

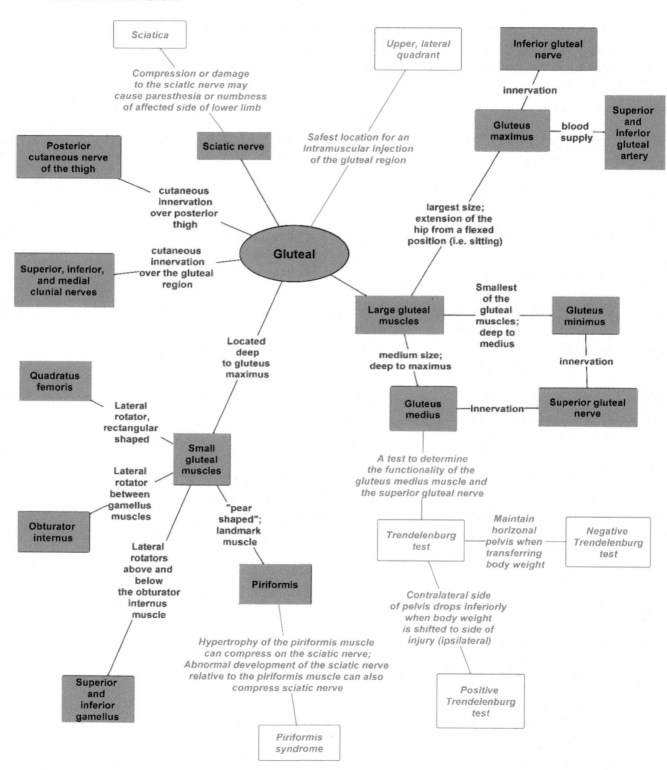

Synthesis Exercise: Create a concept map using items from EXERCISE 2-4.

Exercise 2-4

Primary Category	Secondary Categories	Continuations	Clinical Considerations
Gluteal	Large gluteal muscles	Gluteus maximus	Trendelenburg Test
	Small gluteal muscles	Gluteus minimus	Positive Trend. Test
	Superior, medial, and inferior clunial nerves	Gluteus medius	Negative Trend. Test
		Superior gluteal nerve	Sciatica
	Posterior cutaneous nerve of the thigh	Superior and inferior gluteal artery	Upper, lateral quadrant
	Sciatic nerve	Inferior gluteal nerve	
		Piriformis	
		Superior and inferior gamellus	
		Obturator internus	
		Quadratus femoris	

III. Thigh

Overview of key topics for this section:

- Femoral triangle borders and content
- Compartmentalization of the thigh
- Neurovasculature of the thigh
- Gracilis muscle transplant

What is the femoral triangle? What are its contents?

The **femoral triangle** is a unique anatomical region located in the anterior and proximal thigh. This triangle-shaped space is bound inferiorly and laterally by the sartorius muscle, medially by the adductor longus muscle, (medially), and superiorly by the inguinal ligament (**Figure 2-2)**. (The mnemonic, S.A.I.L. uses the first letter of each border [*S*atorius, *A*dductor, *I*nguinal, *L*igament]). From a lateral to medial direction, the contents of the femoral

Figure 2-2

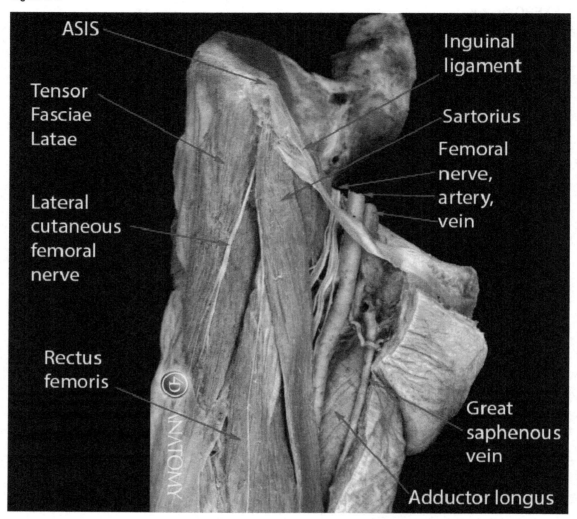

triangle include: 1) the femoral nerve, 2) femoral artery, 3) femoral vein, 4) an empty space with lymphatics. (The learning mnemonic, N.A.V.E.L. uses the first letter of each structure [nerve, artery, vein, empty, lymphatics). A connective tissue sheath called the femoral sheath envelops the femoral artery, femoral vein, and the empty space with lymphatics, but does not include the femoral nerve. Clinically, the femoral artery can be palpated under the skin and used to detect a femoral pulse or insert a catheter. It is found halfway between the **pubic symphysis** and the **anterior superior iliac spine** (ASIS).

How is the thigh compartmentalized?

The thigh region is covered by the **fascia lata**, a stocking-like connective tissue located deep to the subcutaneous fascia. It provides protection and also invests deeper into the thigh as the **intermuscular septum**. The lateral, medial, and posterior intermuscular septum insert onto the linea aspera. As a result, the thigh is divided into anterior, medial, and posterior compartments, which house muscles of similar function and innervation. The **saphenous opening** is a circular opening in the fascia lata near the proximal and antero-medial thigh. The great saphenous vein enters at this location to meet the deeper femoral vein and return superficial venous blood. The **tensor fascia lata** muscle assists withhip and knee joint stability and can tense the IT band and fascia lata during knee extension. It attaches near the ASIS and inserts onto the thickened, lateral aspect of the fascia lata called the **iliotibial (IT) tract** (or band). Its innervation is the superior gluteal nerve.

What provides cutaneous innervation to the thigh?

Cutaneous sensation to the thigh is provided by several nerves. The **lateral cutaneous nerve of the thigh** innervates the lateral thigh region and the **posterior cutaneous nerve of the thigh** innervates the posterior region. The **genitofemoral nerve** innervates the anterior-proximal aspect, and the **anterior cutaneous branches of the femoral nerve** innervate the remaining anterior thigh. The medial thigh is innervated by the **cutaneous branch of the obturator nerve** and the **ilioinguinal nerve**.

How does the anterior compartment of the thigh function?

Hip flexors. The diagonally positioned **sartorius** muscle attaches from the ASIS to the anteromedial aspect of the proximal tibia. It is innervated by the femoral nerve. The **iliopsoas** muscle is the fusion product of the iliacus and psoas major muscles. It attaches from the lumbar vertebral column to the less trochanter of the femur. Upon contraction, the sartorius and iliopsoas flex the hip joint.

    Knee extension. A group of four muscles, known collectively as the **quadriceps**, provides extension of the knee joint. All four muscles, the **vastus intermedius** (deep, middle), **vastus lateralis** (lateral), **vastus medialis** (medial), and **rectus femoris** (superficial, middle) attach to the to the patella bone via the quadriceps tendon, and to the tibial tuberosity via the patellar tendon. The **femoral nerve** supplies all muscles of the anterior compartment and branches as the **saphenous nerve,** which provides cutaneous innervation to the anterior and medial leg.

How does the medial compartment of the thigh function?

Muscles of the medial compartment primarily attach to the pubic bone, ischium, and shaft of the femur. Collectively, the **adductor magnus, adductor longus, adductor brevis, pectineus**, and **gracilis** muscles provide adduction to the lower limb. The adductor magnus is further divided based on functionality. For example, an adductor part can alone flex at hip (via the obturator nerve) and a hamstring part can alone can extend at the thigh (via the tibial part of sciatic nerve). The **obturator externus,** located in the medial compartment allows lateral rotation and adduction. Most of these muscles are innervated by the **obturator nerve** except for the pectineus muscle, which is innervated by the femoral nerve.

How is the gracilis muscle transplanted during surgery?

The gracilis muscle of the medial thigh compartment can be harvested and used as a transplant during surgical operations to improve facial paralysis, anal incontinence, and reconstruction of upper or lower limbs.

How does the posterior compartment of the thigh function?

The muscles of the posterior compartment, or **hamstrings**, include the **biceps femoris** (long and short head), **semitendinosus**, and **semimembranosus.** Collectively, the posterior compartment muscles of the thigh flex at the knee and can extend at the hip following contraction. With the exception of the short head of the biceps femoris, which attaches at the femoral shaft, the proximal attachment of the hamstring muscle is the ischial tuberosity. The distal attachments include the medial tibia (semimembranosus, semitendinosus) and the head of the fibula (biceps femoris). Hamstrings are innervated by the tibial (semimembranosus, semitendinosus, long head biceps femoris) and fibular portions (short head biceps femoris) of the sciatic nerve. The **adductor hiatus** is an opening or passageway in the adductor magnus for the femoral artery and vein to enter the popliteal region.

See CM 2-5A for Review.

CM 2-5A

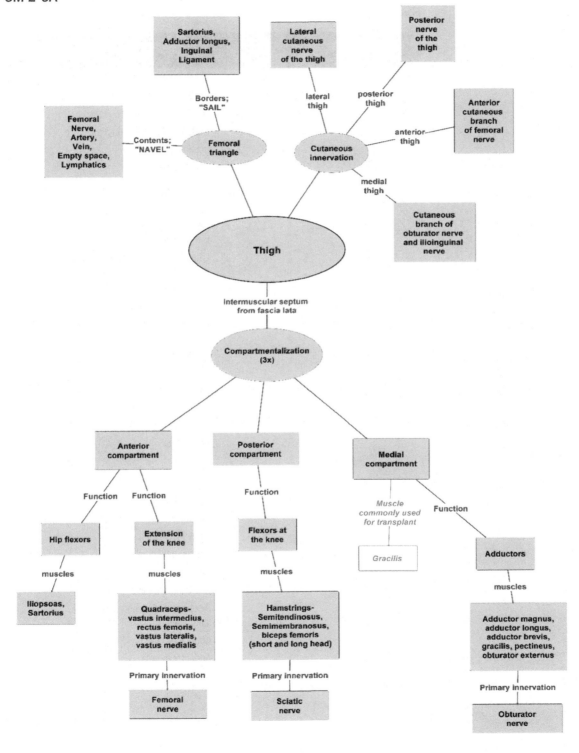

Synthesis Exercise: Create a concept map using items from EXERCISE 2-5.

Exercise 2-5

Primary Category	Secondary Categories	Continuations	Clinical Considerations
Thigh	Femoral triangle	Anterior compartment	Gracilis transplant
	Cutaneous innervation	Posterior compartment	
	Compartmentalization	Medial compartment	
		Sartorius, Adductor longus	
		Inguinal ligament	
		Femoral nerve	
		Femoral artery	
		Femoral vein	
		Empty space	
		Lymphatics	
		Lateral cutaneous nerve of the thigh	
		Posterior nerve of the thigh	
		Anterior cutaneous branch of femoral nerve	
		Cutaneous branch of obturator nerve	
		Ilioinguinal nerve	
		Hip flexors	
		Extension of the knee	
		Flexors of the knee	
		Adductors	
		Iliopsoas	
		Sartorius	
		Vastus intermedius	
		Rectus femoris	
		Vastus lateralis	
		Vastus medialis	
		Semitendinosus,	
		Semimembranosus,	
		Biceps femoris (short and long head)	
		Adductor magnus	
		Adductor longus	
		Adductor brevis	
		Gracilis	

Primary Category	Secondary Categories	Continuations	Clinical Considerations
		Pectineus	
		Obturator externus	
		Femoral nerve	
		Sciatic nerve	
		Obturator nerve	

IV. Knee and Popliteal

Overview of key topics for this section:

- Popliteal fossa region and contents
- Pes anserinus
- Bursitis of the knee

What forms the popliteal fossa ? What are its contents?

The popliteal fossa is a diamond shape located within the posterior aspect of the knee joint. It is a transitional region from the thigh to the leg. The borders include: (1) the semitendinosus and semimembranosus muscles (superomedially), (2) the biceps femoris (superolaterally), and), 3) the medial head of gastrocnemius (inferomedially), and (4) the lateral head of gastrocnemius (inferoaterally), **(see figure 2-3).** Within the popliteal region, the femoral artery and vein enter and gives rise to the popliteal artery and vein. Also, the sciatic nerve is bifurcates here into the fibular and tibial nerves. Venous return from the small saphenous vein to the popliteal vein occurs here as well. The popliteal artery branches into five genicular arteries to supply the knee joint.

What is the pes anserinus?

The pes anserinus (or goose's foot) is a common tendinous attachment on the anterior medial aspect of tibia for the sartorius, gracilis, and semitendinosus muscles. A useful learning mnemonic is S.G.T. (sergeant), representing a letter of each muscle that attaches at the pes anserinus.

Figure 2-3

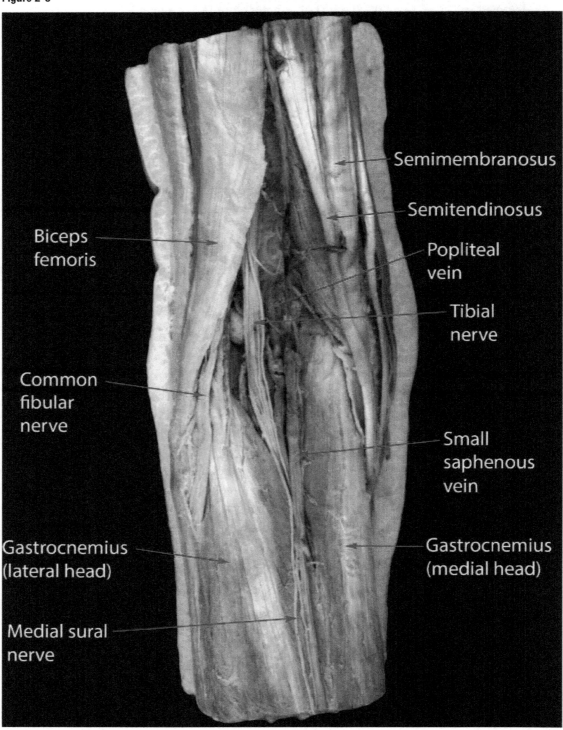

Semimembranosus

Semitendinosus

Popliteal vein

Tibial nerve

Biceps femoris

Common fibular nerve

Small saphenous vein

Gastrocnemius (lateral head)

Gastrocnemius (medial head)

Medial sural nerve

What is bursitis of the knee?

A bursa is a sac like projection within a joint filled with **synovial fluid**. It is typically collapsed but can become irritated or inflamed due to chronic pressure leading to **bursitis**. Bursitis in the knee joint can occur within the **pre-patellar bursa** and the **pes anserinus bursa**.

See CM 2-6A for Review.

CM 2-6A

CHAPTER 2

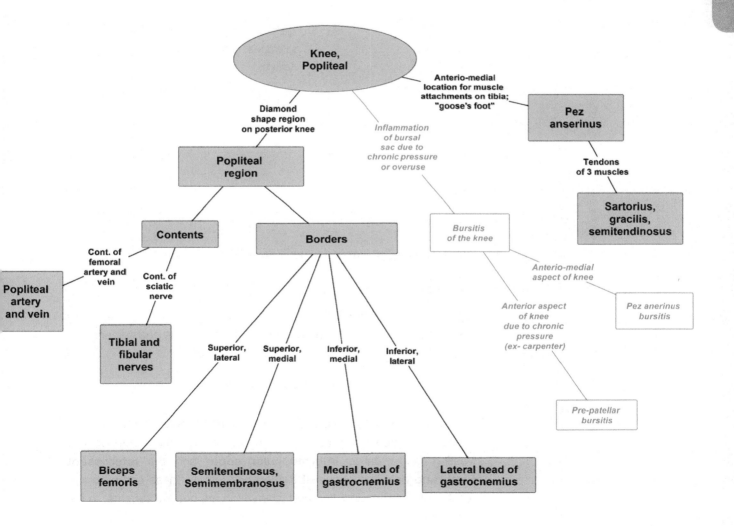

Synthesis Exercise: Create a concept map using items from EXERCISE 2-6.

Exercise 2-6

Primary Category	Secondary Categories	Continuations	Clinical Considerations
Knee, Popliteal	Popliteal region	Borders	Bursitis of the knee
	Pez anserinus	Contents	Pez anserinus bursitis
		Popliteal artery and vein	Pre-patellar bursitis
		Tibial and fibular nerves	
		Biceps femoris	
		Semitendinosus Semimembranosus	
		Medial head of gastrocnemius	
		Lateral head of gastrocnemius	
		Sartorius	
		Gracilis	
		Semitendinosus	

V. Leg

Overview of key topics for this section:

- Compartmentalization of the leg
- Neurovasculature of the leg
- Compartment syndrome and pulse of the dorsalis pedis artery

How is the leg compartmentalized?

The leg is covered by deep fascia called **crural fascia** which help divide the leg into three compartments: anterior, lateral, and posterior. Deep investing fascia called **intermuscular septa** and the **interosseous membrane** between bones of the leg help create these compartments. Muscles of common function and innervation are housed together in each compartment.

What provides cutaneous innervation to the leg?

The **saphenous nerve** is a continuation of the femoral nerve and provides cutaneous innervation to the anteromedial aspect of the leg. The lateral and medial **sural nerves** branch from the **common fibular** and **tibial nerve**, respectively, to innervate the lateral and posterior aspects of the leg.

How does the anterior compartment of the leg function?

Main functions of the anterior compartment of the leg include ankle dorsiflexion and inversion and extension of the digits. During the swing phase of the gait cycle, this compartment becomes active to elevate the foot providing clearance from the ground surface. The **deep fibular nerve,** which branches from the common fibular nerve, innervates anterior compartment muscles. Upon coursing through the interosseous membrane, the **anterior tibial artery** supplies this compartment. The **tibialis anterior** (TA) muscle lies anterior and just lateral to the tibial shaft; it can invert and dorsiflex at the ankle. Distal attachments include the medial cuneiform and first metatarsal bones in the foot. The **extensor hallucis longus (EHL)** muscle is deep and attaches distally to the 1st digit. It primarily extends the 1st digit and assists in dorsiflex of the ankle. The **extensor digitorum longus (EDL)** muscle is located lateral to the TA and attaches to digits 2–5. Similar to the EHL, it primarily extends digits 2–5 and assists in dorsiflexion. The **fibularis tertius** muscle attaches distally to the 5th metatarsal. It can evert and dorsiflex the ankle.

How does the lateral compartment of the leg function?

The lateral compartment of the leg mainly functions to evert the ankle and becomes active during the gait cycle if the ground surface is not level and requires lateral angling of the foot. Innervation includes the **superficial fibular nerve,** which branches from the common fibular nerve. The lateral compartment does not have a true arterial supply, but does receive blood from minor arterioles and capillaries originating from the fibular artery of the posterior compartment. Each tendon from the lateral compartment courses just posterior to the **lateral malleolus** of the ankle to promote eversion. The **fibularis (peroneus) longus** muscle, like the tibialis anterior, attaches distally to the first 1st metatarsal and the medial cuneiform. The **fibularis (peroneus) brevis** muscle, like the fibularis tertius, attaches to the 5th metatarsal and thus, is shorter than the fibularis longus.

How does the posterior compartment of the leg function?

The posterior compartment of the leg has a superficial and a deep compartment, separated by a deep investing fascia. The superficial compartment houses the **triceps surae** which includes the (1) the **gastrocnemius**, (2) **soleus**, and (3) **plantaris** muscles. These muscles fuse distally and attach to the **calcaneus bone** via the **calcaneal tendon (Achilles) (see).** The tibial nerve innervates and the posterior tibial artery and fibular artery supply blood to this the muscles of the superficial compartment. Together, this complex of muscles function to plantarflex the ankle during the push off phase of the gait cycle. The deep compartment includes the (1) **tibialis posterior**, (2) **flexor digitorum longus**, (3) **flexor hallucis longus**, and (4) **popliteus** muscles. The tibialis posterior inserts on the **navicular** and medial cuneiform. The flexor digitorum longus inserts on and flexes digits 2–5. The flexor hallucis longus inserts on, and flexes digit 1. The popliteus muscle lies deep on posterior aspect of the knee joint and helps unlock the knee by slightly rotating the femur laterally by approximately 5 degrees. Similar to the deep compartment, the tibial nerve innervates and the posterior tibial and fibular arteries supply blood to the deep compartment.

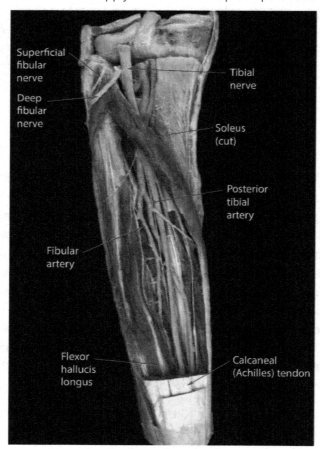

Superficial fibular nerve

Deep fibular nerve

Tibial nerve

Soleus (cut)

Posterior tibial artery

Fibular artery

Flexor hallucis longus

Calcaneal (Achilles) tendon

What is compartment syndrome of the leg? What is the significance of a pulse via the dorsalis pedis artery?

Trauma (e.g., a soccer kick to the anterior compartment or motorcycle accident) can cause compartment syndrome of the leg. Ensuing inflammation can often promote edema (swelling) within an injured compartment. If severe enough, the edema can compress arterial supply and innervation to distal regions such as the foot. The **dorsalis pedis artery** is a continuation of the anterior tibial artery and can be occluded during anterior compartment syndrome. If a pulse is not palpated in the dorsalis pedis artery of the patient, then arterial flow to the dorsum of the foot is likely inhibited.

See CM 2-7A for Review.

CM 2-7A

Synthesis Exercise: Create a concept map using items from EXERCISE 2-7.

Exercise 2-7

Primary Category	Secondary Categories	Continuations	Clinical Considerations
Leg	Anterior compartment	Dorsi flexion	Compartment syndrome
	Posterior compartment	Extension of the digits	Loss of pulse from the dorsalis pedis artery
	Lateral compartment	Eversion	Dorsum of foot
		Superficial compartment	
		Deep compartment	
		Eversion	
		Tibialis anterior	
		Extensor hallucis longus	
		Extensor digitorum longus	
		Fibularis tertius	
		Triceps surae	
		Gastrocnemius	
		Solues	
		Plantaris	
		Tibialis posterior	
		Flexor hallucis longus	
		Flexior digitorum longus	
		Popliteus	
		No true blood supply	
		Capillaries from fibular artery	
		Superficial fibular nerve	
		Deep fibular nerve	
		Posterior tibial artery	
		Fibular artery	
		Tibial nerve	

VI. Ankle, Foot, and Digits

Overview of key topics for this section:

- Medial and lateral malleolus of the ankle
- Cutaneous innervation of foot

- Intrinsic muscles of the foot
- Neurovasculature of the foot
- Tibial nerve entrapment
- Plantar fasciitis

What muscular tendons and neurovasculature course just posterior to the medial malleolus of the ankle? To the lateral malleolus?

Tendons and neurovasculature from the tibilialis posterior, flexor digitorum longus, posterior tibial artery, tibial nerve, and flexor hallucis longus lay just posterior to the medial malleolus. A learning mnemonic for this relationship (anterior to posterior) is **_T_om, _D_ick, _AN_d _H_arry** represents a first letter in the name each structure (**see figure 2-5**). Tendons of the fibularis longus and brevis are located just posterior to the lateral malleolus.

What provides cutaneous innervation to the foot?

The dorsal surface of the foot receives cutaneous innervation mostly from the **superficial fibular nerve**. However, the **deep fibular nerve** supplies a small area of skin between digits 1 and 2 and the **sural nerve** supplies

Figure 2-5

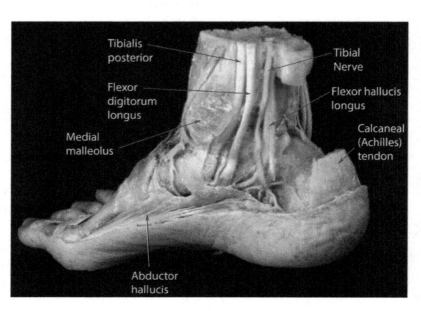

another small region on the lateral aspect of the dorsal foot. Branching from the tibial nerve, the **medial plantar** and **lateral plantar** nerves innervate the respective parts of the plantar surface of the foot. A **medial calcaneal branch** from the tibial nerve provides innervation to the heel of the foot.

What are the four plantar layers in the foot? What muscles are found in each layer? What is the function and innervation for each?

The deep fascia of the plantar foot is called the **plantar fascia**. A very thick part of the plantar fascia is located centrally and called the **plantar aponeurosis.** It protects the deeper muscles and neurovasculature. It is innervated by the **medial calcaneal nerve.** Deep to the aponeurosis, the first true layer of the plantar foot includes has three muscles, each named for the action provided to the foot: the **abductor hallucis** (AH; abducts digit 1), the **flexor digitorum brevis** (FDB; flex digits 2–5), and the **abductor digiti minimi** (ADM; abduct digit 5) muscles (**Figure 2-6).** The medial plantar (AH, FDB) and lateral plantar (ADM) nerves supply these muscles.

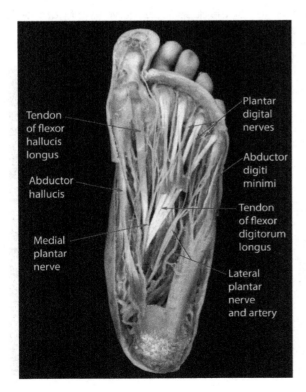

Figure 2-6

Tendon of flexor hallucis longus

Abductor hallucis

Medial plantar nerve

Plantar digital nerves

Abductor digiti minimi

Tendon of flexor digitorum longus

Lateral plantar nerve and artery

The second layer includes the four **lumbricals** (flex digits 2–5 at the proximal interphalangeal joint) and **quadratus plantae** (straightens flexor digitorum longus) muscles, innervated by the medial plantar (single medial lumbrical) and the lateral plantar (lateral 3 lumbricals, quadratus plantae) nerves. In the 3rd layer, we find the **flexor hallucis brevis** (FHB; flexes digit 1), the **adductor hallucis** (AH- oblique and transverse heads; adducts digit 1), and **flexor digiti minimi** (FDM; flexes digit 5). The medial plantar (FHB) and lateral plantar (AH, FDM) supply these muscles. In the 4th layer, the lateral planar nerve innervates the four **dorsal interossei** (DI; adduction of digits) and the three **plantar interossei** (PI; abduction of digits) muscles. Learning mnemonics for associating these muscles and their functions are **PAD** (**P**lantar **AD**duction) and **DAB** (**D**orsal-**AB**duction).

What are the two intrinsic muscles of the dorsal foot? What is the function and innervation for each?

The dorsal foot includes two intrinsic muscles, the **extensor digitorum brevis** (EDB; extends digits 2–5) and the **extensor hallucis brevis** (EHB; extends digit 1), both innervated by the deep fibular nerve (see **figure 2-7).**

Figure 2-7

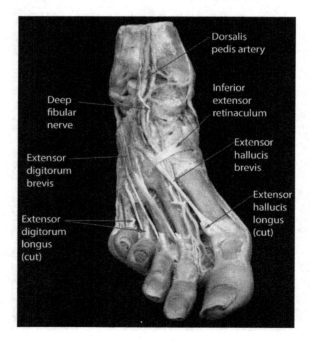

- Dorsalis pedis artery
- Deep fibular nerve
- Inferior extensor retinaculum
- Extensor digitorum brevis
- Extensor hallucis brevis
- Extensor digitorum longus (cut)
- Extensor hallucis longus (cut)

What is tibial nerve entrapment?

Tibial nerve entrapment (or tarsal tunnel syndrome) can occur when distal tendons of the posterior leg compartment compress the tibial nerve as it passes posterior to the medial malleolus, causing numbness, pain, or both. Many possible causal factors are being evaluated, including swelling of tendons, angle of the ankle, and sporting activity.

What is plantar fasciitis?

Plantar fasciitis, or jogger's heal, can occur in avid runners and others. The stimulus is likely a chronic overuse injury, which promotes inflammation, scarring, and breakdown of the plantar fascia at the proximal insertion site. Risk factors include age, weight, physical inactivity, and overuse.

See CM 2-8A and 2-8B for review.

CM 2-8A

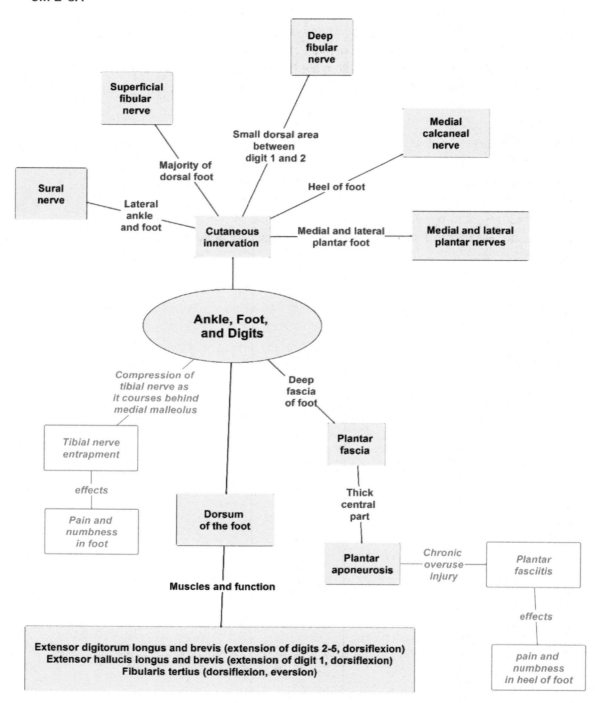

CM 2-8B

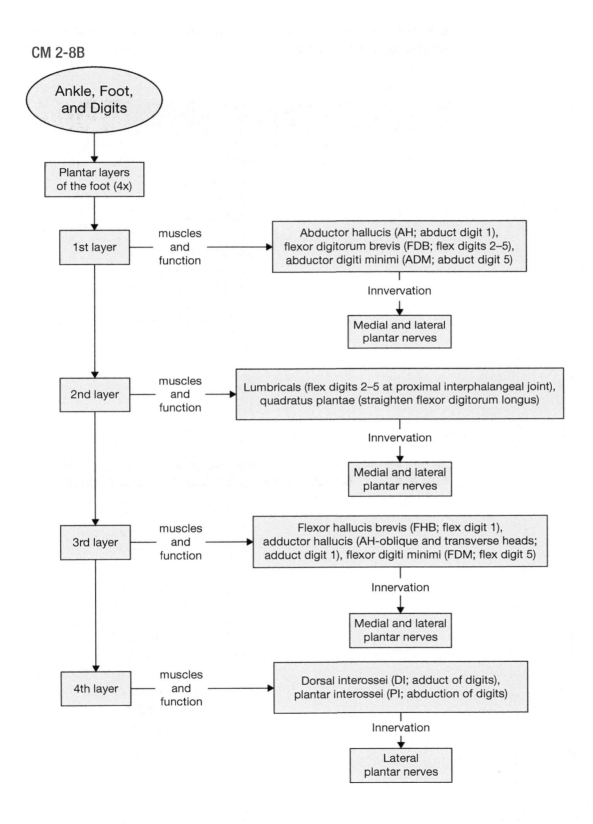

Synthesis Exercise: Create a concept map using items from EXERCISE 2-8A and 2-8B.

Exercise 2-8A

Primary Category	Secondary Categories	Continuations	Clinical Considerations
Ankle, foot, and digits	Cutaneous innervation	Sural nerve	Plantar fasciitis
	Plantar fascia	Superficial fibular nerve	Numbness and pain in heel of foot
	Dorsum of the foot	Deep fibular nerve	Tibial nerve entrapment
		Medial calcaneal nerve	Numbness and pain in the foot
		Medial plantar nerve	
		Lateral plantar nerve	
		Plantar aponeuorsis	
		Extensor digitorum longus and brevis (extension of digits 2–5, dorsiflexion)	
		Extensor hallucis longus and brevis (extension of digit 1, dorsiflexion)	
		Fibularis tertius (dorsiflexion, eversion)	

Exercise 2-8B

Primary Category	Secondary Categories	Continuations
Ankle, foot, and digits	Plantar layers of the foot	Abductor hallucis
		Abduct digit 1
		flexor digitorum brevis
		Flex digits 2–5
		abductor digiti minimi
		Abduct digit 5
		Lumbricals
		Flex digits 2–5 at proximal interphalangeal joint
		Quadratus plantae
		Straighten flexor digitorum longus
		Flexor hallucis brevis
		Flex digit 1
		Adductor hallucis

Primary Category	Secondary Categories	Continuations
		Oblique and transverse heads
		Adduct digit 1
		Flexor digiti minimi
		Flex digit 5
		Dorsal interossei
		Adduct of digits
		Plantar interossei
		Abduction of digits
		Medial plantar nerve
		Lateral plantar nerves

Quick Summary: The Lower Limb as a "Working Model"

Overview of key topics for this section:

- Basic phases of gait
- Specific difference between walking and running gait
- Basic muscle contractions and innervations during each phase of gait

What are the two main phases of gait?

Gait is the pattern of limb movement during locomotion and includes two basic phases.

Phases of Gait

1 **stance phase:** This phase supports the weight of body during contact with the ground surface. It begins with a heel strike and ends with a push off via the forefoot.

2 **swing phase:** During this phase the lower limb makes an anterior movement and has no contact with the ground surface It begins after push off, when the digits leave the ground, and ends when the heal strikes the ground.

What are the specific differences between walking and running gait?

During walking gait, the stance phase occurs approximately 60% of total gait time, and the swing phase includes the remaining approximately 40%. Alterations in both double support (two feet on the ground) and single support (one foot on the ground) occur during walking gait. In contrast, running gait does not have double support, and stance phase is significantly reduced to 20–30% of total gait time while swing phase increases to 70–80%.

Review the basic muscles and nerves required for each phase of gait.

Stance Phase

1 knee extensors accept body weight (rectus femorus; femoral nerve)

2 hip abductors maintain a level pelvis (gluteus medius; superior gluteal nerve)

3 plantar flexors push off the ground (gastrocnemius, soleus; tibial nerve)

Swing Phase

1 hip flexors move the thigh anteriorly (iliopsoas; L1-L3),

2 knee extensors move the leg anteriorly (rectus femoris; femoral nerve),

3 ankle dorsiflexors clear the foot of the ground surface (anterior compartment muscles of the leg; deep fibular nerve)

Image Credits

- Fig. 2-1: Copyright © 2016 by 4D Anatomy. Reprinted with permission.
- Fig. 2-2: Copyright © 2016 by 4D Anatomy. Reprinted with permission.
- Fig. 2-3: Copyright © 2016 by 4D Anatomy. Reprinted with permission.
- Fig. 2-4: Copyright © 2016 by 4D Anatomy. Reprinted with permission.
- Fig. 2-5: Copyright © 2016 by 4D Anatomy. Reprinted with permission.
- Fig. 2-6: Copyright © 2016 by 4D Anatomy. Reprinted with permission.
- Fig. 2-7: Copyright © 2016 by 4D Anatomy. Reprinted with permission.

Chapter 3

Upper Limb

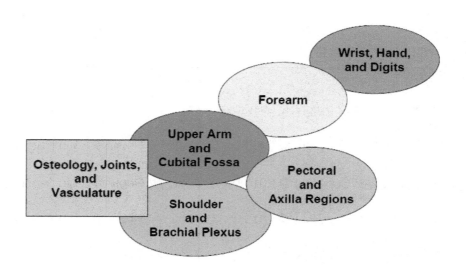

Brief Introduction

What are the basic regions of the upper limb? Consider the deltoid, pectoral, scapular, arm, forearm, wrist, palmar hand, dorsal hand, and digits.

The **shoulder** consists of a transitional site that includes joints of the scapula, clavicle, and humerus. The **deltoid region** is a muscular region located in the proximal upper limb. The **axilla** is lateral to the pectoral region and is often referred to as the arm pit. It is bordered primarily by the **pectoralis**

major muscle anteriorly, and the latissimus dorsi muscle posteriorly. The posterior scapular region contains the scapula. More distally, the **upper arm (**brachial**)** includes a single bone, the humerus, which transitions to the forearm via the elbow joint. The **cubital fossa** resides in the anterior aspect of the elbow, and serves as an important site of phlebotomy (blood draw). The **forearm** (or antebrachial**)** lies distal to the elbow joint and proximal to the wrist. It contains two bones: the radius and ulna. The **wrist** (or carpal) articulates with the **hand**. The **digits** extend directly from the hand. From the anatomical position, the posterior aspect of the hand is dorsum and the anterior is palmar.

I. Osteology, Joints, and Vasculature

Overview of topics for this section:

- Ball and socket joint
- Fractured clavicle
- Shoulder replacement
- Structural Support for the upper arm and forearm
- Fractured humerus and nerves at risk
- Lateral epicondylitis
- Tommy John surgery
- Nursemaid's elbow
- Structural support in the wrist, hand, and digits
- Scaphoid bone fracture
- Boxer's fracture
- Arterial supply to the upper limb and scapula
- High bifurcation of the brachial artery
- Venous drainage of the upper limb
- Phlebotomy

The shoulder joint is a "ball and socket" and includes a wide range of motion. What underlying osteology enables this? What other joints help transition and stabilize the shoulder to the upper limb?

Shoulder. The shoulder joint allows a dynamic range of motion, including circumduction (e.g., a baseball or cricket pitcher). The scapular head is a lateral projection of the scapula and houses the **glenoid cavity** or fossa, which articulates with the head of the humerus. A **supraglenoid** and **infraglenoid** tubercles are located above and below the glenoid fossa, respectively. The **coracoid process** of the scapula is an anterior attachment site for muscles and the **acromion** is a lateral continuation of the scapular spine. The **subscapular fossa** is the anterior flat surface of the scapula. The scapula is stabilized by the **clavicle** (or collar bone). Medially, the clavicle articulates with the **manubrium of the sternum** and creates the **sternoclavicular** (SC) joint. A **sternoclavicular ligament** and **articular disc** made of fibrocartilage help maintain this **saddle-type joint**. The planar-type **acromioclavicular** (AC) joint is created by the lateral end of the clavicle and the acromion. Ligaments also attach from the coracoid process to the clavicle as **coracoclavicular ligaments**. Posteriorly, the scapular spine separates the **supraspinous** and **infraspinous fossas** on the scapula. The humoral head and the glenoid fossa of the scapula form a **ball and socket joint**, called the **glenohumoral joint**. The **glenoid labrum** attaches to the rim of the glenoid fossa to help deepen the joint. Thickenings of the **articular capsule** (or joint capsule) are called **glenohumoral ligaments**. These include superior, middle, and inferior ligaments, which provide stability and prevent dislocation of the shoulder. Articular cartilage lines the humoral head and glenoid fossa to reduce friction between these two bones.

What can cause a fractured clavicle?

The clavicle is S-shaped rather than straight. It serves as a strut which bridges the scapula and sternum. If excessive force is applied during an impact (e.g., falling on shoulder during football tackle), a fracture of the clavicle can occur. Symptoms may include the following: (1) depressed shoulder due to the pull of gravity, (2) medially rotated upper limb due to the pull of pectoralis major muscle, and (3) the medial aspect of clavicle may appear elevated due to the pull of sternocleidomastoid muscle.

What is a shoulder replacement?

Articular cartilage of the glenohumeral joint can become diseased due to osteoarthritis (i.e. overuse or aging). During total shoulder replacement surgery, the head of humerus is removed and replaced with a prosthesis. Also, a new polyethylene cup replaces the diseased portion of the glenoid fossa. Collectively, the new shoulder should improve functionality and reduce pain.

What is the main source of structural support for the upper arm? For the forearm? What unique bony features help translate movements in these regions?

Upper Arm. The proximal aspect of the humerus bone includes the **greater and lesser tubercles,** which create a site of attachment for the rotator cuff muscles (more detail provided later). An **intertubercular groove** resides between the tubercles, through which the long head tendon of the biceps brachii pass. On the posterior shaft of the humerus, the radial nerve courses through the **radial groove**. On the distal aspect of the humerus, medial and lateral epicondyles provide an attachment site for muscles of the forearm. The **capitulum** (lateral) and **trochlea,** (medial) slightly distal to the humeral epicondyles, help establish the elbow joint. The **olecranon fossa** on the posterior humerus accepts the **olecranon** of the ulna from the forearm. Thus, the elbow joint is described as a hinge joint which allows flexion (i.e., decreased angle) and extension (i.e., increased angle).

 Elbow Joint and Forearm. The radius (lateral) and ulna (medial) are located in the forearm. In addition to the hinge joint of the elbow, a pivot joint is created by the **proximal radio-ulnar joint**. It allows **supination** (palm facing anteriorly) and **pronation** (palm facing posteriorly) of the forearm. The head of the radius articulates with the radial notch of the ulna to establish this joint. For stability of the elbow joint, 3 bands (anterior, posterior, oblique) of the **ulnar collateral ligament** (UCL) attach from the medial epicondyle of the humerus to the proximal ulna. Similarly, the **radial collateral ligament** attaches to the lateral epicondyle of the humerus and blends with the **annular ligament**. The radial head is enclosed within the annular ligament and helps maintain the proximal radio-ulnar joint. A **distal radio-ulnar joint** also helps promote supination-pronation of the forearm. The distal radius articulates with the lunate and scaphoid bones of the wrist. However, the ulna does not typically participate in the wrist joint. A styloid process (or spike formation) is found on the very distal aspect of the radius and ulnar.

What can cause a fractured humerus? What nerves are at risk for injury?

Excessive force distributed through the arm can potentially fracture the humerus (e.g., blunt-force trauma or falling on outstretched upper limb). The learning mnemonic, *A.R.M.*, describes common peripheral nerves which are at high risk for injury. A = represents the **axillary nerve** during proximal fracture, R = represents the radial nerve during distal fracture, and M = represents the radial nerve during **mid-shaft fracture**.

What commonly causes pain on the lateral aspect of the elbow joint in avid tennis players or golfers?

Athletes who participate in repetitive extension movements of the wrist, such as a tennis racket swing, can develop lateral epicondylitis (i.e., tennis or golfer's elbow). Overuse of the forearm extensor muscles that attach to the lateral epicondyles can promote inflammation of these tendons (or epicondylitis).

What is an ulnar collateral ligament (UCL) injury? What is Tommy John surgery?

High speed accelerations of the elbow, such as during baseball pitching, can injure the UCL. In 1974, the first major league baseball pitcher to have corrective surgery for this injury was Tommy John. The damaged

UCL can be corrected through reinforcement with an alternative tendon, such as the palmaris longus or patellar tendon. It is surgically woven via a figure 8 fashion into the pre-existing UCL to help re-attain previous performance levels.

What is a subluxation of the radial head (i.e. nursemaid's elbow)?

Also known as nursemaid's elbow, the radial head is prone to subluxation during forces that pull the radius distally, such as playfully swinging a child by their upper limbs. Often, correction of nursemaid's elbow occurs by flexion of the elbow and supination-pronation of the forearm. This movement can guide the radial head back into the annular ligament.

What is a Colles fracture?

Excessive force applied through the wrist (i.e. falling on an out stretched hand) can produce a fracture of the distal radius called Colles fracture. The distal 2 cm of the radius usually project posteriorly, thus curving the wrist and hand like a dinner fork. This injury is the most common type of forearm fracture.

What bones account for both structural support and dynamic movement of the distal upper limb (e.g. bones of the wrist, digits of the hand)?

Wrist, Hand, and Digits. The carpal region includes eight bones which are aligned in two rows of four bones. The proximal row of bones are named **scaphoid**, **lunate**, **triquetral**, and **pisiform,** from lateral to medial. The distal row of bones are named **trapezium**, **trapezoid**, **capitate**, and **hamate,** lateral to medial. Using the first letter of each proximal row bone, lateral to medial, and the reverse order for the distal row produces the mnemonic, *So Long To Pinky, Here Comes The Thumb,* that helps recall each bone. The **distal radial ulnar joint** mainly participates in pronation and

CHAPTER 3

supination of the forearm. Articulation of the scaphoid and lunate bones with the distal radius established the proximal wrist joint, called the **radio-carpal joint**. Five metacarpal bones of the hand articulate with the distal row of carpal bones. These articulation sites are called **carpo-metacarpal joints**. Bones of the digits are called **phalanges** (a total of 14). Digit 1 (thumb) is most lateral and digit 5 (pinky) is most medial within the anatomical position. Each digit has three phalangeal bones (proximal, middle, and distal) with the exception of digit 1 (proximal, distal). The **metacarpal-phalangeal (MCP)** joint is located between the metacarpal and proximal phalanges. The **proximal interphalangeal joint (PIP)** is between the proximal and middle phalanges. Similarly, the **distal interphalangeal joint (DIP)** is between the middle and distal phalanges.

What is a scaphoid bone fracture?

While falling on an out stretched hand with an abducted wrist, the scaphoid is one of the most commonly fractured wrist bones. If the blood supply is damaged, avascular necrosis of the proximal fragment of this bone may also occur, which can promote degenerative joint disease of the wrist later in life.

What is a boxer's fracture?

Excessive force applied to a clenched fist can result in a common injury called boxer's fracture (e.g., boxing competition). The source of fracture is often the neck of the metacarpal bone(s), commonly involving the 5th metacarpal.

What arteries supply the upper limb and scapula?

Arterial Supply to Shoulder. The **subclavian artery** arises from the **brachiocephalic trunk** of the aorta. The **thyrocervical artery** is a short branch from the subclavian and typically gives rise to the **suprascapular and dorsal scapular arteries** (origins may vary). The subclavian artery then courses under the clavicle and continues as the **axillary artery** in three parts. The 1st part courses from the lateral side of the clavicle to the medial border of the pectoralis minor muscle, and includes the superior thoracic artery to supply the first intercostal space. The 2nd part resides deep to the pectoralis minor. It provides branches to the **lateral thoracic artery** and the **thoracoacromial artery,** the latter of which has four branches, one each to the pectoralis muscles, the deltoid, the clavicular regions, and the acromion. Finally, the 3rd part runs from the lateral border of the pectoralis minor to the inferior border of the teres major muscle. Branches of this part include the subscapular artery (branches to the circumflex scapular, thoracodorsal arteries) to the scapular region and circumflex humoral arteries (posterior, anterior) to the deltoid region. Collectively, the brachial plexus, axillary artery, and axillary vein are enveloped in tough connective tissue for protection called the **axillary sheath**.

Arterial Supply to Arm. Distal to the border of the teres major, the axillary artery continues as the **brachial artery**, which courses via the medial aspect of the arm. A **deep brachial artery** (or profunda brachii) branches from the brachial artery and is a main supplier to the muscles of the arm. Also, **ulnar collateral arteries** branch to supply the elbow joint.

Arterial Supply to Forearm. After coursing through the cubital fossa, the brachial artery bifurcates into the **ulnar** and **radial arteries** of the forearm. Branches from these two arteries include the **radial and ulnar recurrent arteries,** which helps supply the elbow joint. A **common interosseous artery** typically branches from the proximal ulnar artery. This immediately splits to create an **anterior and posterior interosseous artery,** which supply the deep anterior and posterior compartments of the forearm, respectively.

Arterial Supply to Wrist, Hand, Digits, The radial artery passes through the **anatomical snuff box** on the lateral and dorsal wrist. It then courses around the posterior aspect of the first digit (thumb) to enter the palm of the hand. It also branches to form the **princeps pollicis artery** of the digit 1 (thumb) and **radialis indicis artery** of the digit 2 (index finger). The ulnar artery enters the wrist and palm via the medial side. Within the palm, these two arteries contribute to form two arterial networks called the **superficial palmar** and **deep palmar arches**. Arising from the superficial palmar arch, the **common palmar digital arteries** split to form the **proper palmar digital arteries, which** supply blood to the medial and lateral aspects of the digits. The deep palmar arch helps supply the deep muscles of the hand.

What is high bifurcation of the brachial artery?

The brachial artery typically bifurcates into the radial and ulnar arteries just distal to the cubital fossa. However, when in rare cases, the bifurcation occurs near the proximal humerus, it is referred to as **high bifurcation** of the brachial artery.

What drains venous blood from the upper limb?

Venous Drainage of the Upper Limb. The venous system of the upper limb has many similarities to the arterial system, including an axillary vein, brachial vein, ulnar and radial veins, palmar venous arches, and digital veins. However, the **cephalic and basilic veins** are unique and maintain a superficial location. The cephalic vein courses between the anterior border of the deltoid and the superior border of the pectoralis major. It continues over the lateral aspect of the upper limb (in the anatomical position). The basilic vein courses over the medial aspect of the upper limb. A **median cubital vein** is quite superficial and connects these two veins within the cubital fossa. Deeper veins accompany the arterial supply such as the brachial and deep artery of the arm. Venous return for the upper limb ultimately leads to the subclavian vein.

What vein is commonly accessed for phlebotomy (blood draw)?

Venous blood samples are generally collected from the median cubital vein during phlebotomy. A tourniquet is placed around the mid-arm to reduce venous return, which increases accessibility for the phlebotomist.

See CM 3-1A, 3-1B, 3-1C, 3-2A, 3-2B, 3-2C, and CM 3-3A for Review.

CHAPTER 3

CM 3-1A

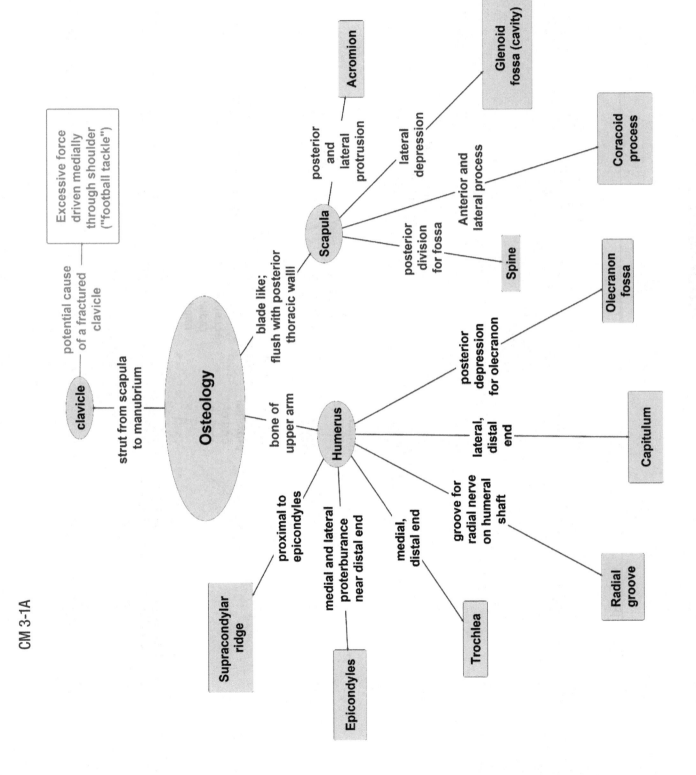

CM 3-1B

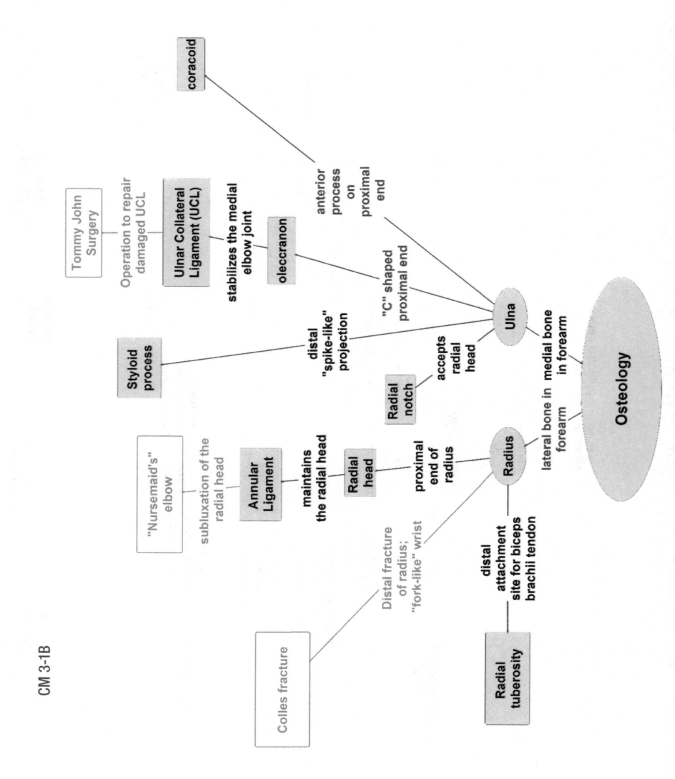

Osteology

- **Ulna** — medial bone in forearm
  - "C" shaped proximal end
    - anterior process on proximal end → coracoid
    - oleccranon
    - Ulnar Collateral Ligament (UCL) — stabilizes the medial elbow joint → Tommy John Surgery — Operation to repair damaged UCL
  - distal "spike-like" projection → Styloid process
  - accepts radial head → Radial notch

- **Radius** — lateral bone in forearm
  - proximal end of radius
    - Radial head — maintains the radial head → Annular Ligament → "Nursemaid's" elbow — subluxation of the radial head
  - distal attachment site for biceps brachii tendon → Radial tuberosity
  - Distal fracture of radius; "fork-like" wrist → Colles fracture

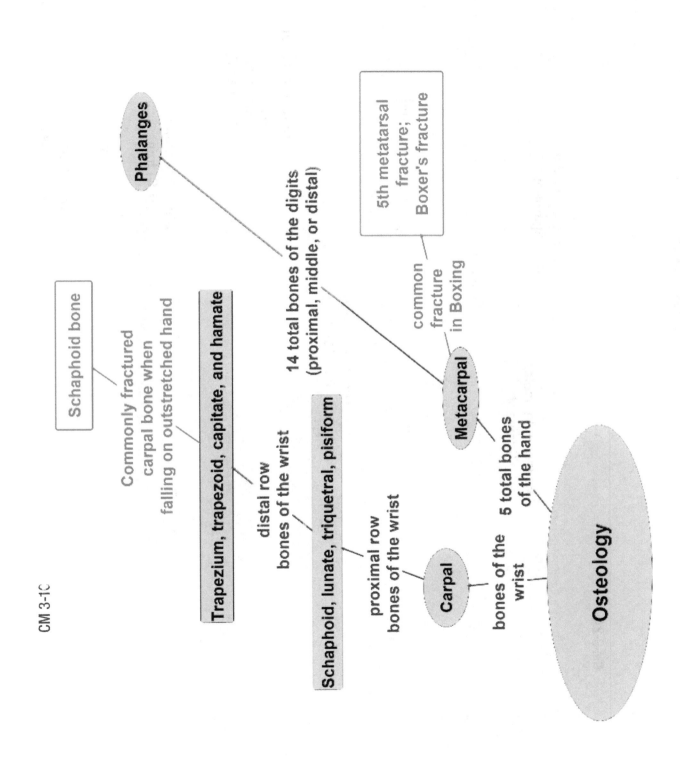

CM 3-10

Phalanges

Schaphoid bone

Commonly fractured
carpal bone when
falling on outstretched hand

Trapezium, trapezoid, capitate, and hamate

distal row
bones of the wrist

14 total bones of the digits
(proximal, middle, or distal)

5th metatarsal
fracture;
Boxer's fracture

common
fracture
in Boxing

Metacarpal

Schaphoid, lunate, triquetral, pisiform

proximal row
bones of the wrist

Carpal

bones of the
wrist

5 total bones
of the hand

Osteology

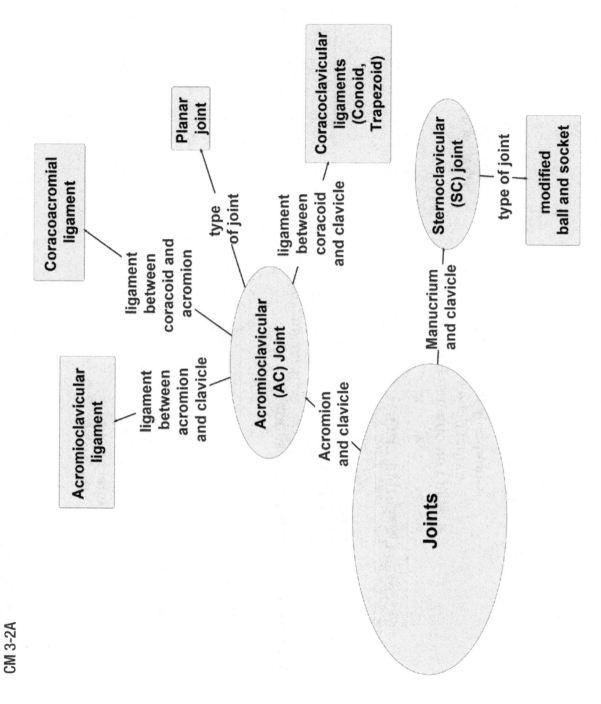

CM 3-2A

CM 3-2B

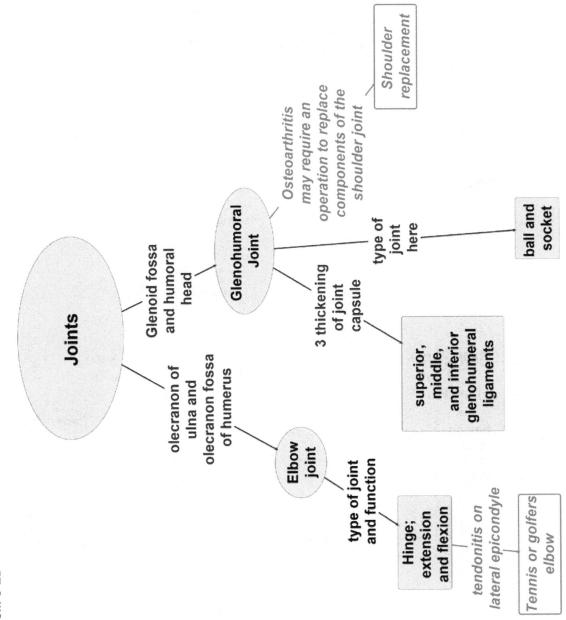

CHAPTER 3

CM 3-2C

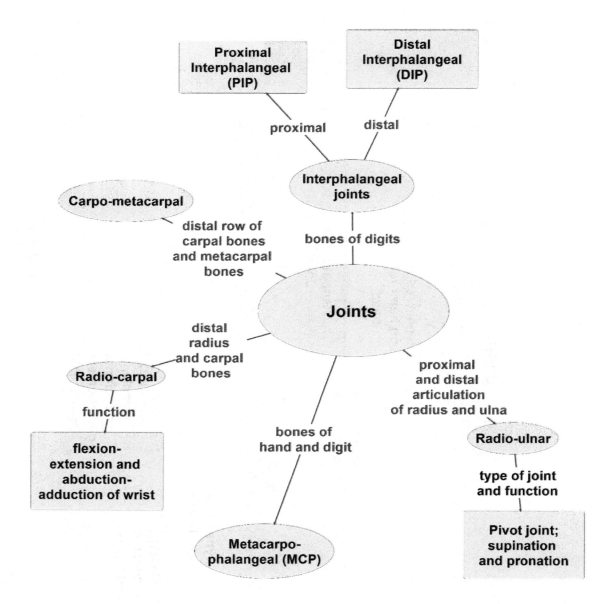

CM 3-3

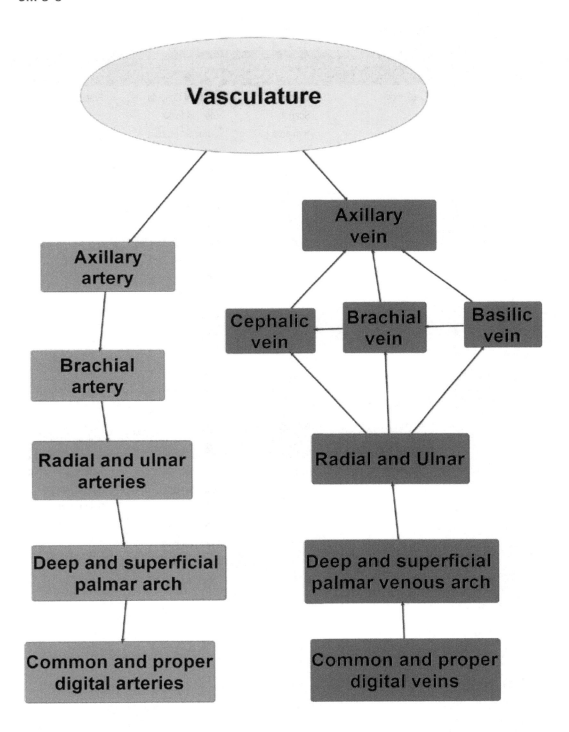

Synthesis Exercise: Create a concept map using items from EXERCISE 3-1A, 3-1B, 3-1C, 3-2A, 3-2B, 3-2C, and 3-3.

Exercise 3-1A

Primary Category	Secondary Categories	Continuations	Clinical Considerations
Osteology	Clavicle	Spine of Scapula	Fractured clavicle
	Scapula	Glenoid fossa	
	Humerus	Coracoid process	
		Acromion	
		Head of humerus	
		Anatomical neck	
		Surgical neck	
		Radial groove	
		Supracondylar ridge	
		Epicondyles	
		Trochlea	
		Capitulum	
		Olecranon Fossa	
		Olecranon	

Exercise 3-1B

Primary Category	Secondary Categories	Continuations	Clinical Considerations
Osteology	Radius	Radial tuberosity	Tommy John Surgery
	Ulna	Radial head	Colles fracture
	Carpal	Radial notch	Nursemaid's elbow
		Annular ligament	
		Styloid process	
		UCL	
		Coracoid process	

Exercise 3-1C

Primary Category	Secondary Categories	Continuations	Clinical Considerations
Osteology	Carpal	Schaphoid	Boxer's fracture
	Metacarpal	Lunate	Schaphoid fracture
	Phalanges	Triquetral	
		Pisiform	
		Trapezium	
		Trapezoid	
		Capitate	
		Hamate	
		Phalanges	

Exercise 3-2A

Primary Category	Secondary Categories	Continuations
Joints	SC joint	AC ligament
	AC joint	Coracoacromial ligament
		Planar joint
		Coracoclavicular ligament
		Modified ball and socket joint

Exercise 3-2B

Primary Category	Secondary Categories	Continuations	Clinical Considerations
Joints	Glenohumoral joint	Ball and Socket joint (true)	Tennis or Golfers Elbow
	Elbow Joint	Sup, Middle, Inf glenohumoral ligament	Shoulder replacement
		Hinge joint; Flexion-extension	

CHAPTER 3

Exercise 3-2C

Primary Category	Secondary Categories	Continuations
Joints	Radio-ulnar joint	Pivot joint; Supination, pronation
	Radio-carpal joint	Supination, pronation
	Carpo-metacarpal joint	Flexion-extension ;Abduction-Adduction
	MCP joint	PIP joint
	IP Joints	DIP joint
		Hinge joint

Exercise 3-3

Primary Category	Arterial	Venous
Vasculature	Axillary	Axillary
	Brachial	Brachial
	Radial	Cephalic
	Ulnar	Basilic
	Deep Arch	Radial
	Superficial Arch	Ulnar
	Common Digital	Deep Arch
	Proper Digital	Superficial Arch
		Common Digital
		Proper Digital

II. Shoulder and Brachial Plexus

Overview of topics for this section:

- Scapulohumoral muscles of the shoulder
- Rotator cuff tear and repair
- The brachial plexus
- Upper and lower brachial plexus injuries

What are the scapulohumoral muscles of the shoulder? What muscles are considered rotator cuff muscles? How are these muscles innervated and supplied with blood?

Six scapulohumoral muscles cross the shoulder joint: the deltoid, teres major, teres minor, supraspinatus, infraspinatus, and subscapularis. The **deltoid** is the largest and represents approximately 40% of the total scapulohumoral muscle mass. It is divided into three parts that have different proximal attachments. The anterior part attaches to the lateral clavicle and mainly serves to flex the upper arm. The middle part attaches to the acromion and abducts the upper arm. The posterior part attaches to the scapular spine and primarily extends the upper arm. All parts attach distally at a common site of the humerus called the **deltoid tuberosity**. The **axillary nerve** innervates the deltoid and exits posteriorly from the brachial plexus. The **posterior circumflex humoral artery** from the axillary artery and a **deltoid branch** from thoracoacromial artery supply blood.

The **teres major** muscle attaches to the inferior angle of the scapula and the medial lip of the intertubercular groove of the humerus. Similar to the latissimus dorsi, it assists with adduction and medial rotation of the upper limb. Innervation and blood supply are via the lower subscapular nerve and circumflex scapular artery, respectively.

A family of four rotator cuff muscles includes the supraspinatus, infraspinatus, teres minor, and subscapularis (or **S.I.T.S**). Together, these muscles secure the head of the humerus in the glenohumeral joint and assist in movements at the shoulder. The **supraspinatus** attaches from the **supraspinous fossa** of the scapula to the greater tubercle of the humerus. Upon contraction, it initiates the first 15° of abduction. The **infraspinatus** attaches from the infraspinatus fossa to the greater tubercle. It helps laterally rotate the upper limb. The suprascapular nerve and artery supply the supra- and infraspinatus muscles. The **teres minor** attaches from the lateral and inferior aspect of the **infraspinous fossa** to the greater tubercle. It provides adduction and lateral rotation. The axillary nerve also innervate the teres minor. The **subscapularis** attaches from the subscapular fossa to the lesser tubercle, and medially rotates the upper limb. The upper and lower subscapular nerves innervate this muscle.

Figure 3-1A

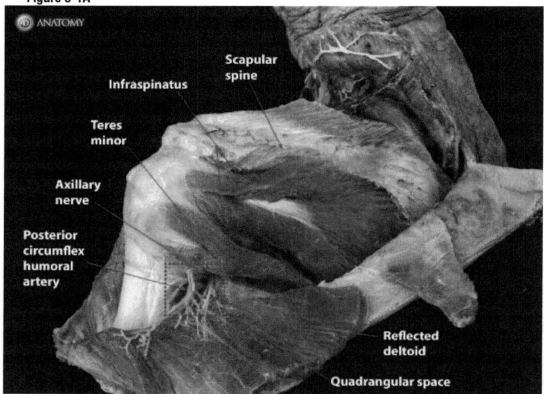

Figure 3-1B

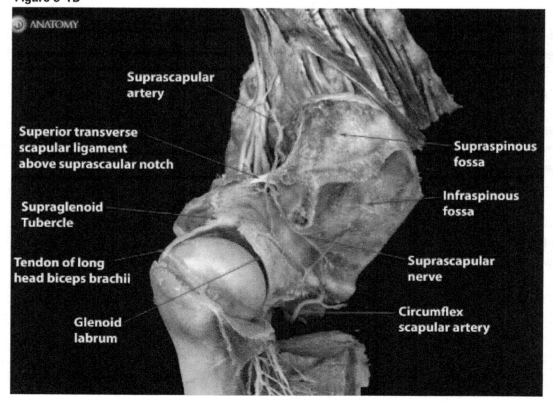

What is a rotator cuff tear? How does tendonitis of the supraspinatus muscle occur? How does surgery repair and improve this condition?

Chronic overuse or excessive strain (e.g., baseball pitching) can tear tendons of the muscles crossing the shoulder joint. Also, if the subacromial space does not provide sufficient space for the supraspinatus tendon, the repetitive movements of tendon against the acromion may cause inflammation (or tendonitis). Repair of a torn supraspinatus tendon and improvement of the subacromial space can be accomplished surgically.

What is the brachial plexus (provide both a simple and an advanced description)? Where is it located? What peripheral nerves are produced from the brachial plexus?

The **brachial plexus** is a network of nerves originating from spinal segments C5–T1 that ultimately help innervate the upper limb. From proximal to distal, its structure includes roots, trunks, divisions, cords, and peripheral nerves. The ventral (anterior) primary rami of C5–T1, or the roots, initially

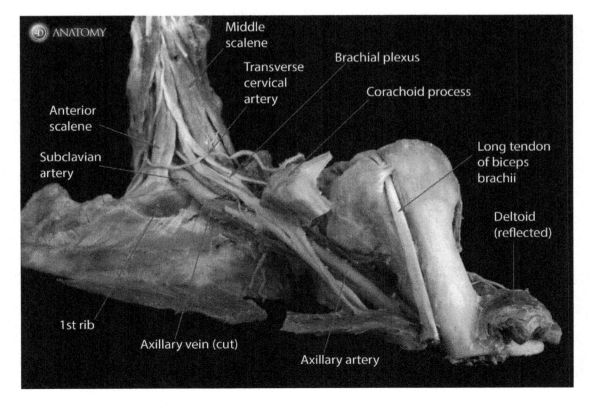

Figure 3-1C

CHAPTER 3

form the brachial plexus and pass between the anterior and middle scalene muscles.

The superior (C5–C6), middle (C7), and inferior trunks (C8–T1) then continue either anteriorly or posteriorly, relative to the axillary artery, designating the anterior and posterior divisions. The lateral cord branches as the musculocutaneous nerve and also contributes to the median nerve. The medial cord gives rise to the ulnar nerve and also makes a contribution to the median nerve. The posterior cord branches as the axillary and radial nerves. These peripheral nerves are discussed with more detail in the following sections. Each peripheral nerve receive contributions from multiple spinal nerves. The integration of spinal nerves to produce a single peripheral nerve represents an essential concept for understanding functional deficits associated with brachial plexus injuries.

What functional deficits are associated with upper and lower brachial plexus injuries? What other neuropathies can affect the upper limb?

Erb's palsy. Upper brachial plexus injuries frequently occur when introducing stretch or traction between the neck and shoulder (e.g., falling off a ladder and separating neck and shoulder, or a stretch of newborn's neck during child birth). Damage to the root of C5 and C6 are at risk and can result in Erb's palsy (or waiter's tip). This commonly produces atrophy of the deltoid and weakness of the biceps brachii muscles as well as a medially rotated upper limb at rest. Commonly impacted peripheral nerves are the suprascapular, musculocutaneous, axillary, and long thoracic nerves.

Klumpke's palsy. A lower brachial plexus injury can occur following the introduction of distal stretching to the upper limb (e.g., grabbing a tree branch while falling from a tree, or excessive stretching of the upper limb during childbirth). The roots of C8 and T1 are at risk for injury and may promote Klumpke's palsy, in which a claw like hand presents at rest due to unopposed influence of the forearm extensors. Commonly affected nerves include the median and ulnar nerves.

Winged scapula. Following a long thoracic nerve injury, a dysfunctional serratus anterior muscle causes the scapula to project posteriorly, in a wing like configuration.

Radial neuropathy, or wrist drop syndrome. Damage or trauma to the radial nerve impairs the contraction of forearm extensor muscles, and producing a limp wrist.

Thoracic outlet syndrome. Compression to the neurovasculature, such as the brachial plexus roots or subclavian artery, can promote thoracic outlet syndrome (TOS). Limited space or impingements within the superior outlet can facilitate shooting pain or numbness to the hands, forearm, or arm. Causes of TOS include (1) congenital malformations like a cervical rib or muscular abnormalities; (2) trauma such as whiplash injuries; and (3) localized tumor growth, in rare cases.

See CM 3-4, 3-5A, and 3-5B for Review.

CM 3-4

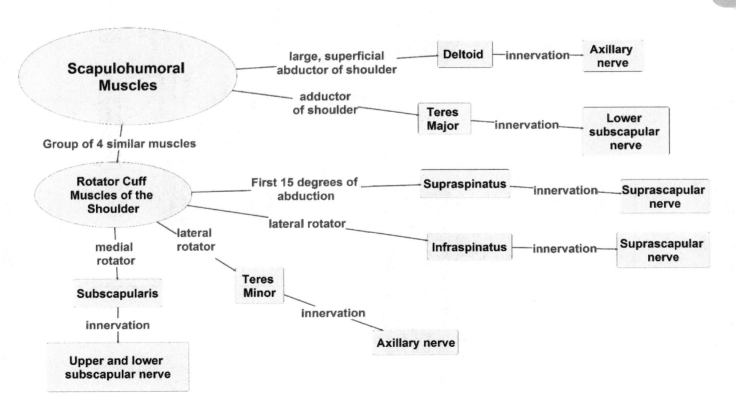

CM 3-5A

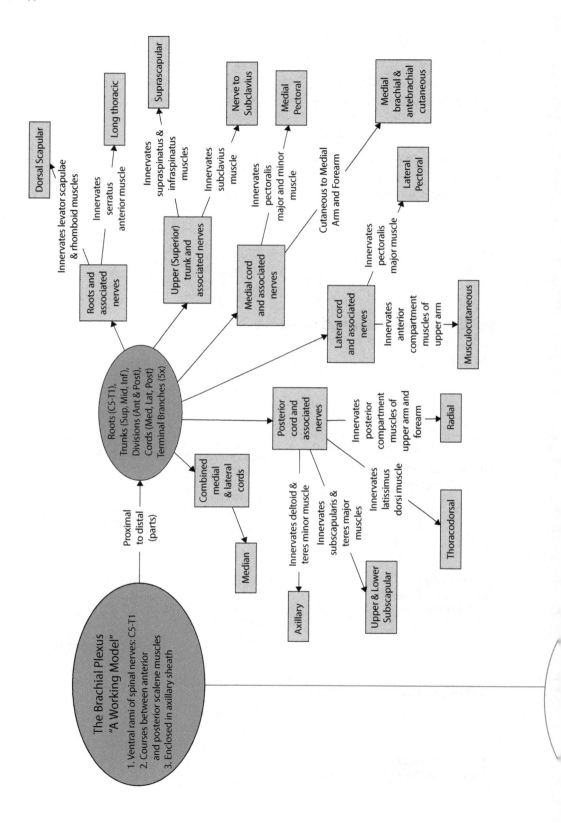

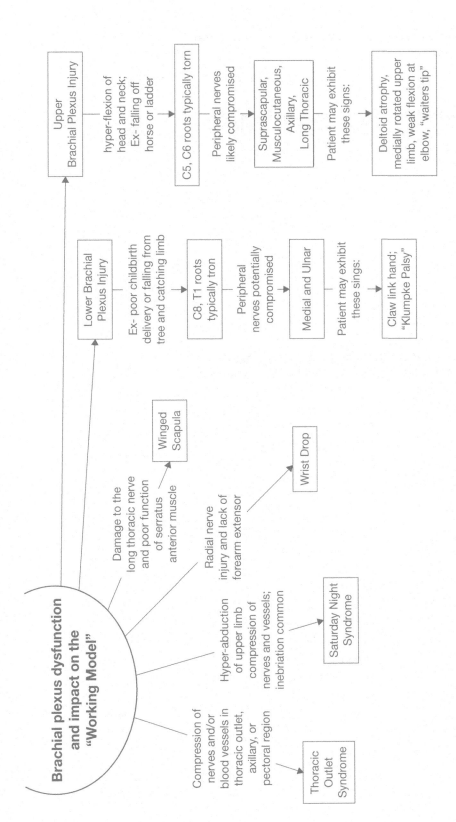

Brachial plexus dysfunction and impact on the "Working Model"

Compression of nerves and/or blood vessels in thoracic outlet, axillary, or pectoral region → Thoracic Outlet Syndrome

Hyper-abduction of upper limb compression of nerves and vessels; inebriation common → Saturday Night Syndrome

Radial nerve injury and lack of forearm extensor → Wrist Drop

Damage to the long thoracic nerve and poor function of serratus anterior muscle → Winged Scapula

Lower Brachial Plexus Injury → Ex- poor childbirth delivery or falling from tree and catching limb → C8, T1 roots typically tron → Peripheral nerves potentially compromised → Medial and Ulnar → Patient may exhibit these sings: → Claw link hand; "Klumpke Palsy"

Upper Brachial Plexus Injury → hyper-flexion of head and neck; Ex- falling off horse or ladder → C5, C6 roots typically torn → Peripheral nerves likely compromised → Suprascapular, Musculocutaneous, Axillary, Long Thoracic → Patient may exhibit these signs: → Deltoid atrophy, medially rotated upper limb, weak flexion at elbow, "waiters tip"

CM 3-5B

Synthesis Exercise: Create a concept map using items from EXERCISE 3-4, 3-5A, and 3-5B.

Exercise 3-4

Primary Category	Secondary Categories	Continuations
Scapulohumoral muscles	Rotator cuff muscles	Subscapularis
	Deltoid	Teres minor
	Teres major	Infraspinatus
		Supraspinatus
		Upper subscapular nerve
		Lower subscapular nerve
		Axillary nerve
		Suprascapular nerve

Exercise 3-5A

Primary Category	Secondary Categories	Continuations
Brachial Plexus	Roots, trunks, divisions, cords, terminal nerves	Roots and associated nerves
		Upper trunk and associated nerves
		Medial cord and associated nerves
		Lateral cord and associated nerves
		Posterior cord and associated nerves
		Combined median and lateral cords
		Median nerve
		Axillary nerve
		Upper & Lower Subscapular nerve
		Thoracodorsal nerve
		Radial nerve
		Musculocutaneous nerve
		Lateral pectoral nerve
		Medial brachial cutaneous nerve
		Medial antebrachial cutaneous nerve
		Medial pectoral nerve
		Nerve to subclavius
		Suprascapular nerve
		Dorsal scapular nerve
		Long thoracic nerve

Exercise 3-5B

Primary Clinical Consideration	Secondary Clinical Considerations	Clinical Continuations
Brachial Plexus Dysfunction	Injury to C5–C6 roots	Injury to C5–C6 roots
	Suprascapular nerve impaired	Suprascapular nerve impaired
	Musculocutaneous nerve impaired	Musculocutaneous nerve impaired
	Axillary nerve impaired	Axillary nerve impaired
	Long thoracic nerve impaired	Long thoracic nerve impaired
	Deltoid atrophy	Deltoid atrophy
	Medially rotated upper limb	Medially rotated upper limb
	Weak flexion at elbow	Weak flexion at elbow
	"Waiters tip"	"Waiters tip"
	Injury to C8-T1 roots	Injury to C8-T1 roots
	Medial nerve impaired	Medial nerve impaired
	Ulnar nerve impaired	Ulnar nerve impaired
	"Claw-like" hand	"Claw-like" hand
	Klumpke Palsy	Klumpke Palsy

III. Pectoral and Axilla Regions

Overview of topics for this section:

- Pectoral muscles
- The axilla

What muscles are located in the pectoral region? How do they produce movements of the upper limb? How are they innervated and supplied with blood?

The **pectoralis major** muscle is a large superficial muscle with proximal attachments to the clavicle (clavicular head), the sternum (sternocostal head), and the abdominal wall (abdominal part). Distally, it attaches to the lateral lip of the intertubercular groove of the humerus. Upon contraction, the

CHAPTER 3

clavicular head flexes at the shoulder joint. The sternoclavicular head can produce an extension movement starting from a flexed position. As a whole, the pectoralis major can also adduct or medially rotate the upper limb. Both the **lateral and medial pectoral nerves** innervate the pectoralis major. The **pectoralis minor** is smaller and deep to the major. It attaches from the coracoid process to ribs 3–5 to stabilize the scapula upon contraction. Innervation is via the **medial pectoral nerve**. The thoracoacromial artery provides pectoral branches, which supply the pectoralis major and minor. The **serratus anterior muscle** attaches from the anteromedial aspect of the scapula and ribs 1–8 (can vary). The long thoracic nerve innervates this muscle, which helps stabilize the scapula via protraction. Blood supply includes the lateral thoracic artery. The **subclavius muscle** is located just inferior to the clavicle and innervated by the nerve to the subclavius. It helps depress the clavicle.

What is the axilla? What are its boundaries?

The **axilla,** or arm pit, is bound by the following borders: (1) anteriorly by the pectoralis major, (2) posteriorly by the latissimus dorsi and teres major, (3) laterally by the humerus, and (4) medially by the serratus anterior and thoracic wall. In addition to the neurovasculature destined for the upper limb, it houses axillary fat, including lymph nodes that drain the upper limb and pectoral region. Deep fasciae named for the muscle they cover include the deltoid fascia, pectoral fascia (for pectoral major), and clavipectoral fascia (covering the pectoralis minor and subclavius muscles) and are continuous with the brachial fascia of the arm.

See CM 3-6A and 3-6B for Review.

CM 3-6A

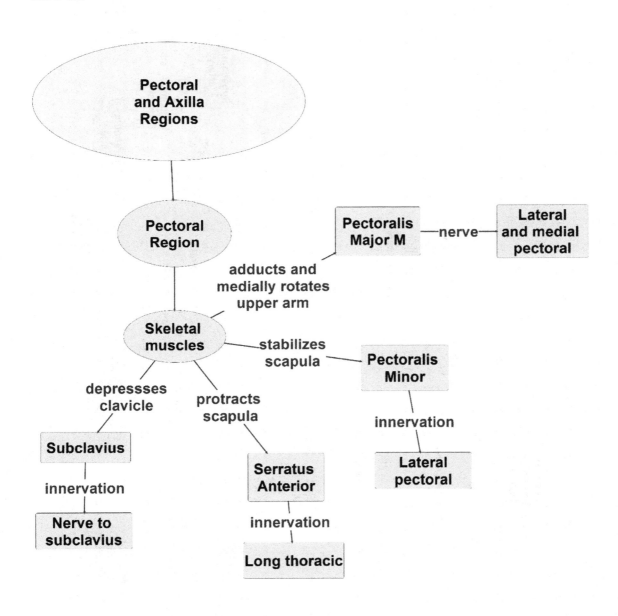

CM 3-6B

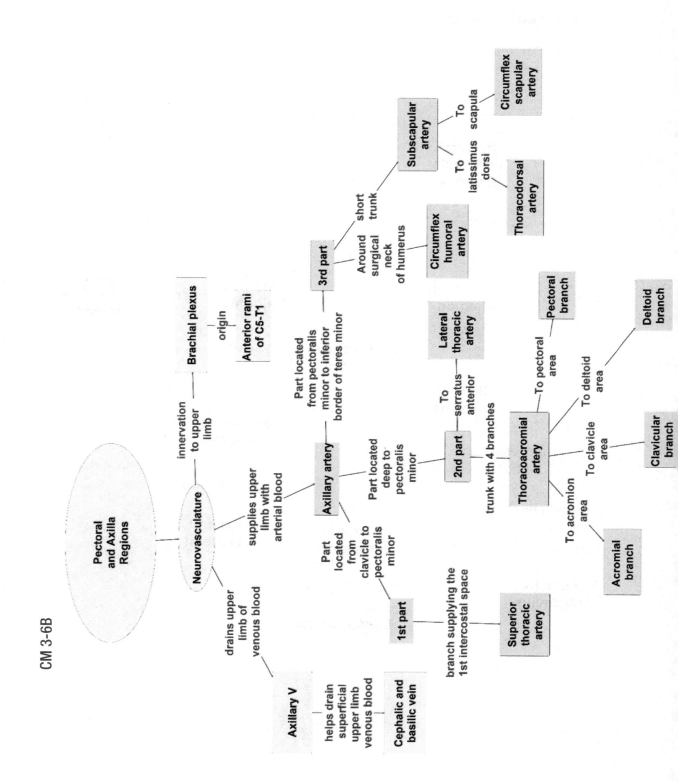

Synthesis Exercise: Create a concept map using items from EXERCISE 3-6A and 3-6B.

Exercise 3-6A

Primary Category	Secondary Categories	Continuations
Pectoral and axilla region	Pectoral region	Skeletal muscles
		Pectoralis major muscle
		Pectoralis minor muscle
		Serratus anterior muscle
		Subclavius muscle
		Lateral pectoral nerve
		Medial pectoral nerve
		Long thoracic nerve
		Nerve to subclavius

Exercise 3-6B

Primary Category	Secondary Categories	Continuations
Pectoral and Axilla region	Neurovasculature	Axillary artery
		Axillary vein
		Cephalic vein
		Basilic vein
		1st part
		2nd part
		3rd part
		Thoracoacromial artery
		Acromial branch
		Clavicular branch
		Deltoid branch
		Pectoral branch
		Circumflex humoral artery
		Subscapular artery
		Thoracodorsal artery
		Circumflex scapular artery
		Superior thoracic artery
		Lateral thoracic artery

IV. Upper Arm and Cubital Fossa

Overview of topics for this section:

- Muscle compartments of the upper arm including muscles, key attachments, nerves, and actions
- The cubital fossa and contents

What muscle compartments are created by deep investing fascia in this region? What muscles are located in each compartment? What common relationships can be established in each compartment regarding actions and innervations?

The **brachial fascia** is superficial and continuous with the deltoid, pectoral, & axillary fasciae. It gives rise to deep investing fasciae, which envelop each muscle. The medial and lateral intramuscular septa establish an anterior and posterior compartment of the arm. Each compartment houses muscles with similar functions, such as flexors or extensors.

The **anterior compartment** includes two flexor muscles of the elbow joint (biceps brachii, brachialis) and a shunt muscle (a muscle that resists dislocation of the joint- **coracobrachialis**) **(Figure 3-2)**. The **biceps brachii** has two heads and is a powerful flexor of the elbow in a supinated position. It also helps supinate the forearm. The short head attaches proximally to the coracoid process. The long head tendon travels through the intertubercular groove to attach at the supraglenoid tubercle. These two muscle bellies fuse distally to attach at the radial tuberosity. The **brachialis muscle** lies deep to the biceps brachii and flexes the elbow in all positions. It attaches from the mid-shaft of the humerus to the coronoid process of the ulna. The coracobrachialis muscle stabilizes the glenohumoral joint. Attachments include the coracoid process and mid-shaft of the humerus. Blood is supplied to the muscles of the arm by the deep artery of the arm (**profundus brachii**), and innervation to the anterior compartment is the **musculocutaneous nerve** (C5–C6[7]).

Figure 3-2

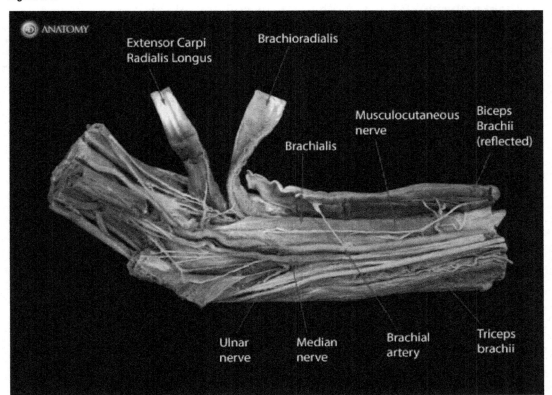

The **posterior compartment** contains one true extensor muscle (triceps brachii) with a medial head (deep), lateral head, and long head (medial, superficial). The **medial head** is considered the most active both with and without major resistance. The **lateral head** is recruited during contractions against high resistance. Similar to the coracobrachialis, the **long head** is a shunt muscle for the shoulder joint. The **radial nerve** (C5 – T1) innervates the triceps brachii. An additional small muscle, the **anconeus**, on the posterior aspect of the elbow joint, helps prevent the elbow joint capsule from being pinched. The ulnar and median nerves travel within the medial arm, but have no major branches in this region.

Where is the cubital fossa? What are the contents of this region?

Within the anterior aspect of the elbow joint is the **cubital fossa (see figure 3-2)**. It resembles a triangular shape created by the brachioradialis (lateral), the pronator teres (medial), and the biceps brachii tendon (an imaginary superior border located between the two humoral epicondyles). The **median cubital vein**, which unites the cephalic and basilic veins, courses over the superficial cubital fossa. A **bicipital aponeurosis** from the biceps brachii covers and protects the deep cubital fossa. From medial to lateral, the median nerve, brachial artery, biceps brachii tendon, and radial nerve pass through the cubital fossa. (A helpful learning mnemonic created from first letters in these structures' names is **My B**lood **T**urns **R**ed). The brachial artery bifurcates immediately distal to this region to help supply the medial (ulnar artery) and lateral (radial artery) forearm. The ulnar nerve does not participate in the cubital fossa since it courses posterior to the medial epicondyle of the humerus, in a groove referred to as the cubital tunnel. Force or compression applied here (e.g., hitting your funny bone) can produce acute pain.

See CM 3-7A and 3-7B for Review.

CM 3-7A

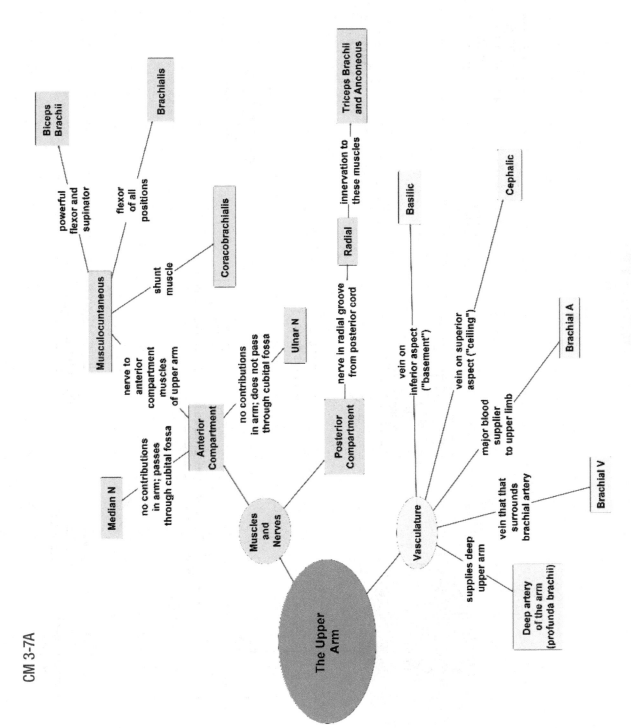

CHAPTER 3

CM 3-7B

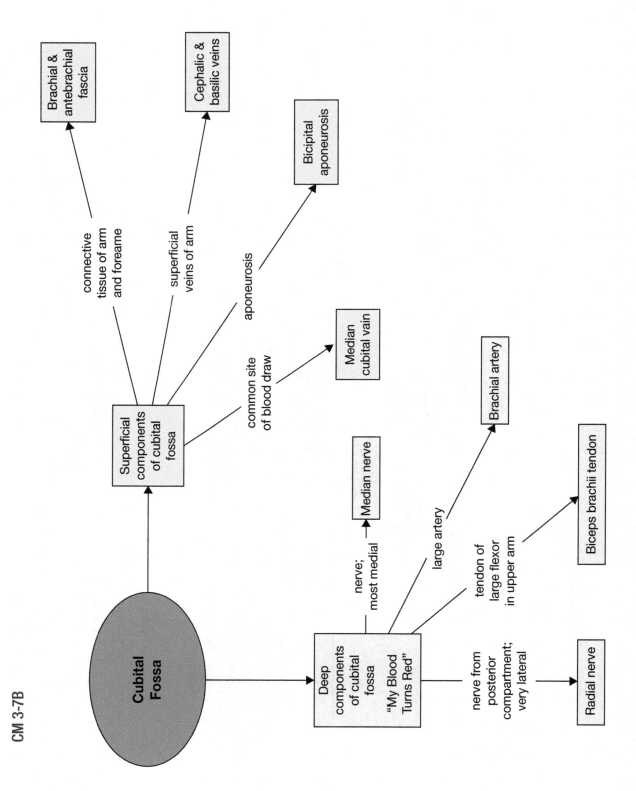

Cubital Fossa

connective tissue of arm and foreame → Brachial & antebrachial fascia

superficial veins of arm → Cephalic & basilic veins

aponeurosis → Bicipital aponeurosis

Superficial components of cubital fossa

common site of blood draw → Median cubital vain

Deep components of cubital fossa "My Blood Turns Red"

nerve; most medial → Median nerve

large artery → Brachial artery

tendon of large flexor in upper arm → Biceps brachii tendon

nerve from posterior compartment; very lateral → Radial nerve

Synthesis Exercise: Create a concept map using items from EXERCISE 3-7A and 3-7B.

Exercise 3-7A

Primary Category	Secondary Categories	Continuations
Upper Arm	Muscles and Nerves	Anterior compartment
	Vasculature	Posterior compartment
		Median nerve
		Musculocutaneous nerve
		Ulnar nerve
		Biceps brachii muscle
		Brachialis muscle
		Coracobrachialis
		Radial nerve
		Triceps brachii muscle
		Anconeous muscle
		Basilic Vein
		Cephalic vein
		Brachial artery
		Brachial vein
		Deep artery of the arm

Exercise 3-7B

Primary Category	Secondary Categories	Continuations
Cubital fossa	Superficial cubital fossa	Brachial fascia
	Deep cubital fossa	Antebrachial fascia
		Cephalic vein
		Basilic vein
		Bicipital aponeurosis
		Median cubital vein
		Median nerve
		Brachial artery
		Biceps brachii tendon
		Radial nerve

V. Forearm

Overview of topics for this section:

- Muscle compartments of the forearm including muscles, key attachments, nerves, and actions

What muscle compartments are created in this region? What muscles are located in each compartment? What common relationships can be established in each compartment regarding actions and innervations? What are the exceptions to these common relationships? What peripheral nerves are involved with cutaneous innervation of the forearm?

The forearm separates into anterior and posterior compartments with the radius, ulnar, and interosseous membrane providing the division. In general, the anterior compartment houses muscles of flexion and pronation and the posterior compartment contains the extensors and supinators. The **antebrachial fascia** is a continuation of the brachial fascia, and surrounds the forearm. Specifically, muscle function of the anterior compartment includes (1) flexion of the elbow, (2) pronation of the forearm, (3) flexion, abduction, and adduction of the wrist, and (4) flexion of the digits. It is arranged in three layers (superficial, middle, deep). The superficial layer includes four muscles, which all attach proximally to the medial epicondyle (**pronator teres, flexor carpi radialis, palmaris longus**, and **flexor carpi ulnaris**). The median nerve innervates each muscle except the flexor carpi ulnaris (ulnar nerve). The middle layer includes a single muscle, the **flexor digitorum superficialis (FDS)**. Its tendons attach at the middle phalange of digits 2–5 and the median nerve also innervates the FDS muscle. A deep muscle layer is composed of three muscles: the **flexor digitorum profundus (FDP), flexor pollicis longus (FPL)**, and **pronator quadratus**. The FDP tendon passes in between FDS tendon just before attaching to the distal phalanges of digits 2–5. The FPL attaches to the distal phalange of digit 1. A very deep pronator quadratus muscle spans the distal radius and ulna. Deep muscles of this compartment are typically innervated by a specific branch of the median nerve called the **anterior interosseous nerve** (C8–T1) except for the medial half of the FDP (ulnar nerve).

Figure 3-3A

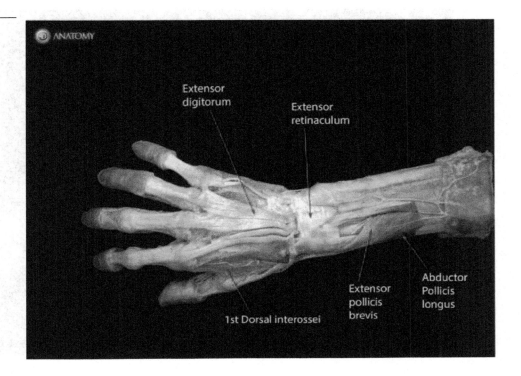

The posterior compartment includes two muscle layers (superficial, deep) which function to (1) extend, abduct, and adduct the wrist; (2) extend the digits; and (3) extend and abduct the thumb. The radial nerve and its deep branch, the **posterior interosseous nerve,** innervates all muscles of the posterior compartment, . The superficial layer is composed of the **brachioradialis, extensor carpi radialis (longus, brevis), extensor digitorum, extensor digiti minimi,** and the **extensor carpi ulnaris** muscles **(see figure 3-3A)**. Although the brachioradialis is considered a posterior compartment muscle, it actually acts as a weak flexor to the elbow. The deep layer muscles consist of the **abductor pollicis longus, extensor pollicis brevis,** and **extensor pollicis longus (see figure 3-3B)**. The extensor indicis acts on digit 2 (index finger) and the supinator muscle creates the floor of the cubital fossa. Long extensor tendons pass under a thick band of the antebrachial fascia, called the **extensor retinaculum,** and helps hold the tendons in place during contractions. The cutaneous innervation of the forearm includes the medial cutaneous nerve of the forearm (medial aspect), the musculocutaneous nerve (lateral aspect), and the posterior cutaneous nerve of the forearm (remaining posterior aspect).

See CM 3-8A and 3-8B for Review.

CHAPTER 3

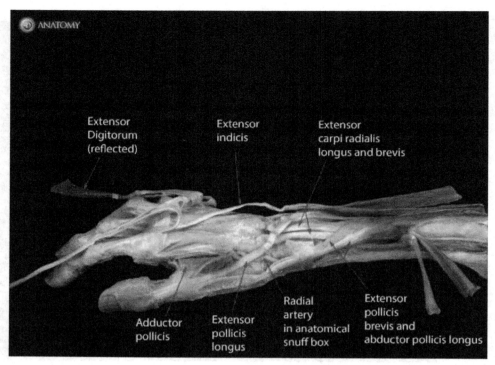

Figure 3-3B

CM 3-8A

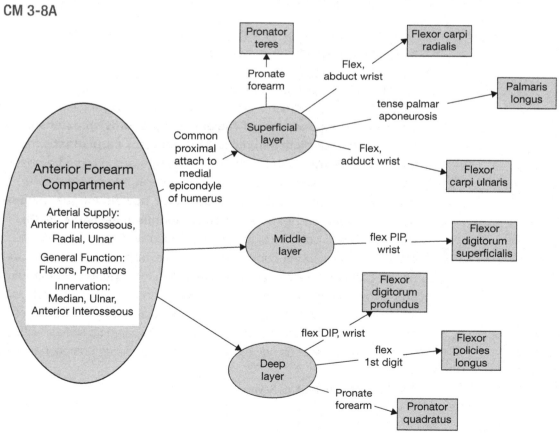

CM 3-8B

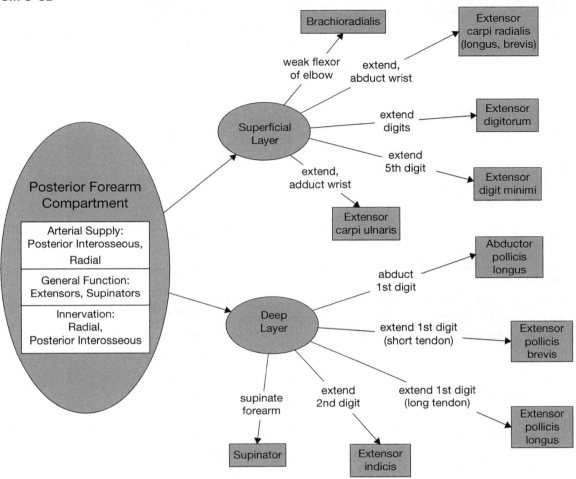

Synthesis Exercise: Create a concept map using items from EXERCISE 3-8A and 3-8B.

Exercise 3-8A

Primary Category	Secondary Categories	Continuations
Anterior Compartment of Forearm	Superficial Layer	Pronotor teres muscle
	Middle Layer	Flexor carpi radialis muscle
	Deep Layer	Palmaris longus muscle
		Flexor carpi ulnaris muscle
		Flexor digitorum superficialis muscle
		Flexor digitorum profundus muscle

Primary Category	Secondary Categories	Continuations
		Flexor pollicus longus muscle
		Pronator quadratus muscle
		Flexion
		Pronation
		Adduction
		Abduction
		Median nerve
		Ulnar nerve
		Anterior interosseous nerve
		Radial artery
		Ulnar artery
		Anterior interosseous artery

Exercise 3-8B

Primary Category	Secondary Categories	Continuations
Posterior Compartment of Forearm	Superficial layer Deep layer	Brachioradialis muscle
		Extensor carpi radialis longus muscle
		Extensor carpi radialis brevis muscle
		Extensor digitorium muscle
		Extensor digiti minimi muscle
		Extensor carpi ulnaris muscle
		Abductor pollicus longus muscle
		Extensor pollicus brevis muscle
		Extensor pollicus longus muscle
		Extensor indicis muscle
		Supinator muscle
		Extension
		Supination
		Abduction
		Adduction
		Radial nerve
		Posterior interosseous nerve
		Radial artery
		Posterior interosseous artery

VI. Wrist, Hand, and Digits

Overview of topics for this section:

- The extensor retinaculum, palmar carpal ligament, and the flexor retinaculum
- Carpal tunnel and contents
- Guyon's canal and contents
- Carpal tunnel syndrome
- Cyclist's palsy
- Palmar aponeurosis, thenar fascia, hypothenar fascia
- Synovial sheath and fibrous sheath of long tendons
- Compartments of the hand including muscles, key attachments, innervations, and actions
- The extensor expansion and the Z movement
- Cutaneous innervation to the hand

What is the difference between the extensor retinaculum, palmar carpal ligament, and flexor retinaculum (transverse carpal ligament)? What is the carpal tunnel? What are its contents? What is Guyon's Canal? Contents?

At the very distal and palmar aspect of the forearm (or carpal region) is a thickening of antebrachial fascia called the **palmar carpal ligament**. The tendons of the flexor digitorum superficialis (FDS) and profundus (FDP) reside deep to this structure and are arranged in sets of 2 × 2 (FDS) and 1 × 4 (FDP). More distally, the carpal bones, the hook of hamate (medial), the tubercle of trapezium (lateral), and the **flexor retinaculum (or transverse carpal ligament)** create the carpal tunnel **(see figures 3-4A, 3-4B)**. Within the carpal tunnel we find the (1) median nerve, (2) FDS (tendons), 3) (FDP (tendons), and (4) flexor pollicis longus tendon (FDL). Also, the FDS and FDP are arranged in sets of 1 × 4 (FDS) and 1 × 4 (FDP) in the carpal tunnel.

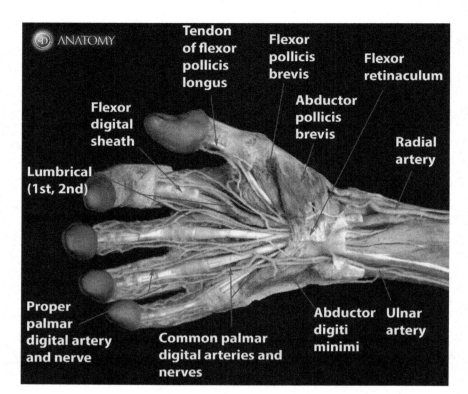

Figure 3-4A

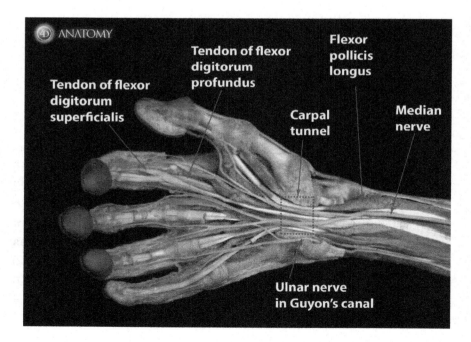

Figure 3-4B

What is Carpal Tunnel Syndrome?

Compression of the median nerve in the carpal tunnel can occur due to inflammation of the long flexor tendons. Potential causes include repetitive overuse of wrist and hand movements (e.g., a computer mouse) or infection. Symptoms include numbness, tingling, and weakness over the lateral ½ of the hand. Proper ergonomics and a wrist brace may help relieve this condition. However, the central palm is unaffected because the palmar cutaneous branch of the median nerve arises before the carpal tunnel.

What is Cyclist's Palsy (handcuff palsy)?

The ulnar canal (Guyon's Canal) is located between the pisiform and hook of hamate bones on the medial wrist (**see figure 3-4B**). The ulnar nerve, which passes through this canal, is often compressed at this location in avid cyclists or from wearing tight handcuffs.

What is the palmar aponeurosis, thenar fascia, and hypothenar fascia?

The antebrachial fascia continues into the palmar hand via three parts: (1) the **palmar aponeurosis** in the central palm, (2) the **thenar fascia** over the lateral palm, and (3) the **hypothenar fascia** over the medial palm. The palmar aponeurosis is very thick and protective. It attaches to the palmaris longus tendon of the forearm.

What allows long tendons of the digits to slide freely? What maintains adherence of the tendons to their respective bones?

Synovial sheaths surround the long flexor tendons to reduce friction and ease sliding with their respective bones. The **ulnar bursa** envelops the FDS and FDP tendons while the **radial bursa** surrounds the FPL tendon. Digital synovial sheaths also surround each digit. The **fibrous sheaths,** such as the annular (circular) and cruciform (cross-like) sheaths, form a protective tunnel that adheres the tendons to the bone.

What are the 4 compartments of the hand? What muscles are found in each compartment? What is the function and innervation of each? What is the extensor expansion and the Z-movement?

The **thenar compartment** resides just proximal and medial to digit 1 (**see figure 3-4A**). It houses three muscles including the abductor pollicis brevis (APB), flexor pollicis brevis (FPB), and the opponens pollicis. Each is named for the respective function acting on digit 1 and is innervated by the recurrent branch of the median nerve.

The **adductor compartment** is located within the deep and lateral aspects of the palm. The adductor pollicis muscle is located here and includes two heads, one oblique (proximal) and one transverse (distal). This muscle is innervated by the ulnar nerve and adducts digit 1.

The **hypothenar compartment** comprises four muscles and is located on the medial palm (**see figure 3-4A**). Three of the four muscles act on digit 5, including the abductor digiti minimi, flexor digiti minimi, and opponens digiti minimi. Each is named for its respective function. The palmaris brevis muscle of this compartment is thought to protect the ulnar artery and nerve at the wrist. The ulnar nerve innervates all muscles of this compartment.

The **central compartment** houses two main sets of muscles including the four lumbricals and the seven interossei (**see figure 3-4A, 3-4B**). The **lumbricals** attach from the tendon of the FDP to the extensor expansion of the extensor digitorum and allows flexion at the MCP joint. Also, simultaneous extension of the digits at the PIP and DIP joints can occur, which is referred to as a **Z movement**. The median nerve innervates the two lateral lumbricals and the ulnar nerve innervates the medial two lumbricals. The interosseous muscles are sub-divided into two groups based on location. The three **palmar interossei** reside in the deep anterior palm and serve to adduct the digits. Four **dorsal interossei** are found in the dorsum of the hand and abduct the digits. (*Note: Using the following learning mnemonic may help differentiate the interossei muscles and function: 1) **P**almar → **AD**duct: **PAD**, 2) **D**orsal → **AB**duct: **DAB***). All interosseous muscles are innervated by the ulnar nerve.

See CM 3-9A for Review.

CM 3-9A

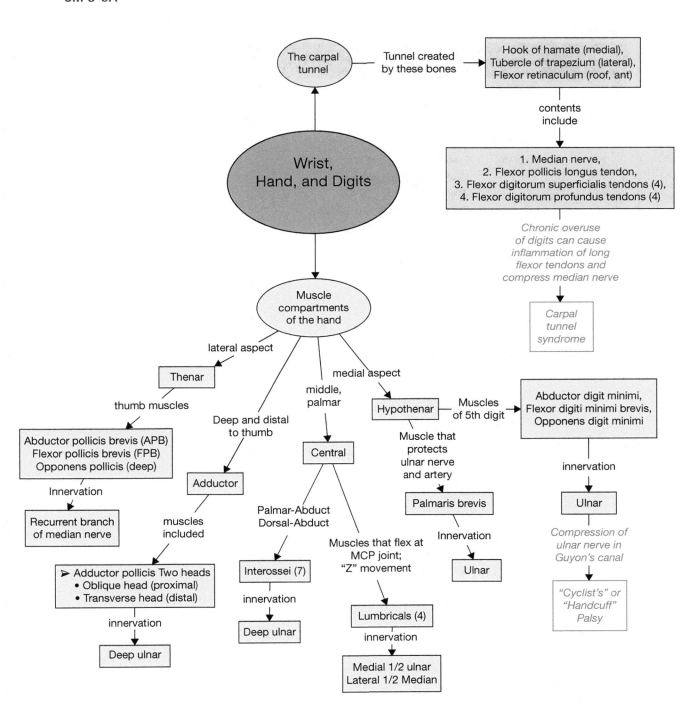

Synthesis Exercise: Create a concept map using items from EXERCISE 3-9.

Exercise 3-9

Primary Category	Secondary Categories	Continuations	Clinical Considerations
Wrist	Carpal tunnel	Hook of Hamate	Carpal tunnel syndrome
Muscle compartments of the hand	Thenar	Tubercle of trapezium	Cyclist's (Handcuff) Palsy
	Central	Flexor retinaculum	
	Hypothenar	Median nerve	
	Adductor	Flexor pollicus longus tendon	
		Flexor digitorum superficialis tendons	
		Flexor digitorum profundus tendons	
		Abductor pollicus brevis muscle	
		Flexor pollicus brevis muscle	
		Opponens pollicus muscle	
		Lumbricals	
		Dorsal interossei muscles	
		Palmar interossei muscles	
		Abductor digiti minimi muscle	
		Flexor digiti minimi muscle	
		Opponens digiti minimi muscle	
		Palmaris brevis	
		Adductor pollicus muscle	
		Deep Ulnar nerve	
		Ulnar nerve	
		Median nerve	
		Recurrent branch of median nerve	
		Flexion	
		Abduction	
		Adduction	
		Opposition	
		"Z" movement	

What nerves provide cutaneous innervation to the hand? What are their territories?

Areas of cutaneous innervation for the hand are distributed among the median nerve (tips, palmar and distal dorsal aspects of digit 1, 2, 3, and half of 4), the radial nerve (dorsal and lateral aspects of hand), and the ulnar nerve (palmar and dorsal aspect of medial hand, medial half of digit 4, all of digit 5).

Quick Summary: The Upper Limb as a Working Model

Use an integrated approach to understand the upper limb as a working model. Review the nerves listed below. Focus on normal upper limb function and predict the functional consequence of injury to each nerve. Consider how the location of nerve injury (proximal, distal) impacts overall functionality.

Upper Limb Nerves

A. *Axillary Nerve* (C5–C6; posterior cord) **(see figure 3-5)**

    1   innervates deltoid, teres minor

    2   superior, lateral branch, cutaneous branch to upper arm

B. *Radial Nerve* (C5–T1; posterior cord) **(see figure 3-5)**

    1   innervates muscles of posterior compartment

    2   therefore, motor component is extension of elbow

    3   continues to forearm (motor & sensory)

    4   runs in the radial groove of humerus

Figure 3-5

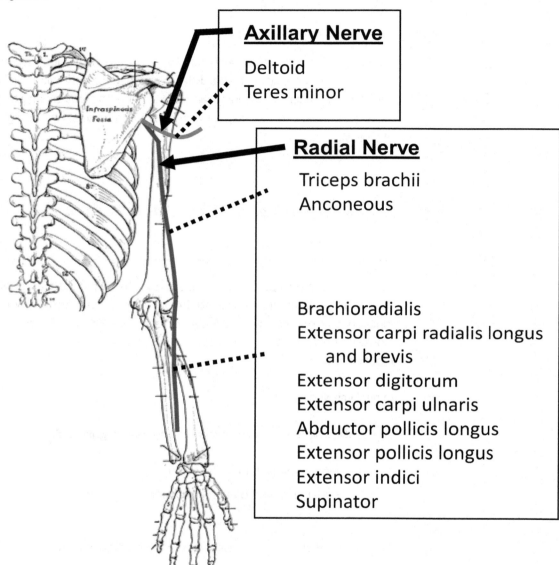

Axillary Nerve

Deltoid
Teres minor

Radial Nerve

Triceps brachii
Anconeous

Brachioradialis
Extensor carpi radialis longus
    and brevis
Extensor digitorum
Extensor carpi ulnaris
Abductor pollicis longus
Extensor pollicis longus
Extensor indici
Supinator

C. *Musculocutaneous Nerve* (C5–C6[7]; lateral cord) **(see figure 3-6)**

    1   innervates muscles of anterior compartment

    2   therefore, motor component involves elbow flexion and forearm supination

    3   sensory component to lateral aspect of forearm

    4   ***pierces coracobrachialis muscle then passes between bicep and brachialis

Figure 3-6

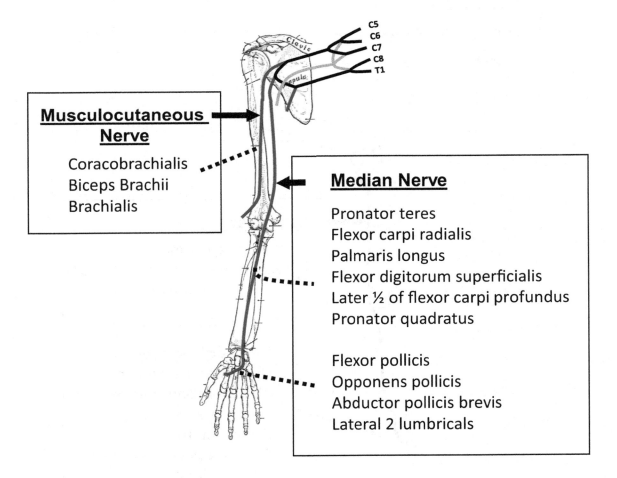

Musculocutaneous Nerve

Coracobrachialis
Biceps Brachii
Brachialis

Median Nerve

Pronator teres
Flexor carpi radialis
Palmaris longus
Flexor digitorum superficialis
Later ½ of flexor carpi profundus
Pronator quadratus

Flexor pollicis
Opponens pollicis
Abductor pollicis brevis
Lateral 2 lumbricals

C5
C6
C7
C8
T1

CHAPTER 3

D. *Median Nerve* (C5–T1; medial and lateral cord) **(see figure 3-6)**

    1   located in the anterior compartment

    2   no branches in the arm

    3   runs anterior to the brachialis and medial to the bicipital tendon in the cubital fossa

E. *Ulnar Nerve* (C[7]8–T1; medial cord) **(see figure 3-7)**

    1   located in the anterior compartment

    2   then pierces the medial intermuscular septum to the posterior compartment, then travels posterior to the medial epicondyle

    3   no major branches in the arm

    4   often referred to as the *funny bone*

Figure 3-7

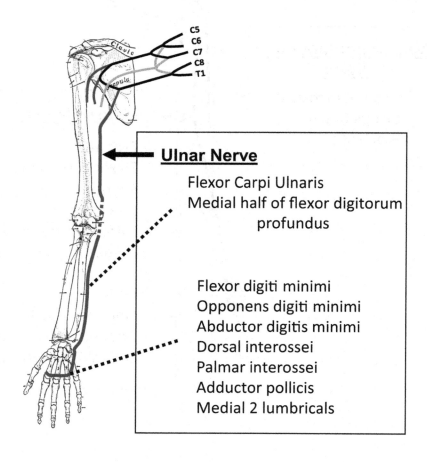

Ulnar Nerve

Flexor Carpi Ulnaris
Medial half of flexor digitorum
profundus

Flexor digiti minimi
Opponens digiti minimi
Abductor digitis minimi
Dorsal interossei
Palmar interossei
Adductor pollicis
Medial 2 lumbricals

Image Credits

- Fig. 3-1A: Copyright © 2016 by 4D Anatomy. Reprinted with permission.
- Fig. 3-1B: Copyright © 2016 by 4D Anatomy. Reprinted with permission.
- Fig. 3-1C: Copyright © 2016 by 4D Anatomy. Reprinted with permission.
- Fig. 3-2: Copyright © 2016 by 4D Anatomy. Reprinted with permission.
- Fig. 3-3A: Copyright © 2016 by 4D Anatomy. Reprinted with permission.
- Fig. 3-3B: Copyright © 2016 by 4D Anatomy. Reprinted with permission.
- Fig. 3-4A: Copyright © 2016 by 4D Anatomy. Reprinted with permission.
- Fig. 3-4B: Copyright © 2016 by 4D Anatomy. Reprinted with permission.
- Fig. 3-5: Adapted from John Charles Boileua Grant, "Axillary And Radial Nerve With Muscles," https://commons.wikimedia.org/wiki/File:Grant_1962_2.png. Copyright in the Public Domain.
- Fig. 3-6: Adapted from John Charles Boileua Grant, "Musculocutaneous and Median Nerve With Muscles," https://commons.wikimedia.org/wiki/File:Grant_1962_1.png. Copyright in the Public Domain.
- Fig. 3-7: Adapted from John Charles Boileua Grant, "Ulnar Nerve With Muscles," https://commons.wikimedia.org/wiki/File:Grant_1962_1.png. Copyright in the Public Domain.

Chapter 4

Neck

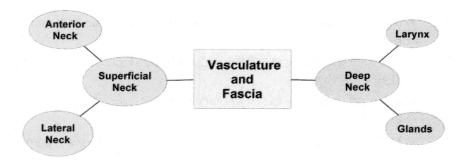

Brief Introduction

What is the neck? What anatomic features are included?

The neck is a transitional region between the head and thorax. It includes major blood vessels, the airway (i.e., larynx, trachea), a digestive tube (i.e., esophagus), cranial nerves (e.g., vagus, facial, hypoglossal), lymph nodes, and glands (e.g., thyroid, parathyroid, submandibular). Several skeletal muscles are located in the posterior neck region for movements of the head (see Chapter 1) and in the anterior neck region for movements of the **hyoid bone** (i.e., **infrahyoid**, **suprahyoid**). Cervical investing fascia also create a variety of compartments in the neck (e.g., pre-tracheal, pre-vertebral, carotid sheath). For osteology and joints of the neck, see Chapter 1.

I. Vasculature and Fasciae

Overview of key topics for this section:

- Carotid artery
- Carotid sinus and body
- Orthostatic hypotension
- Jugular vein
- Cervical fascia and compartments

What are the common carotid, internal carotid, and external carotid arteries? Carotid sinus? Carotid body?

The **common carotid artery** is bilateral and enveloped in a protective, connective tissue called the **carotid sheath (see figure 4-1)**. The right carotid artery typically branches from the brachiocephalic artery and the left from the aortic arch, although variation of their origins occurs. The carotid artery is 6.0–6.5 cm long. At approximately the C4 vertebrae, the common carotid bifurcates into an internal and an external carotid artery. The path of the **internal carotid artery** (ICA) follows a superior direction towards the external opening of the carotid canal of the skull. This opening is just anterior to the jugular foramen. The ICA provides arterial blood to the brain. The **external carotid** artery also directs superiorly, but maintains a more superficial and anterior position relative to the ICA. After coursing just behind the mandible, it supplies the superficial and deep face with arterial blood via several smaller branches.

Located at the bifurcation of the common carotid artery is a collection of specialized chemoreceptor cells, collectively called the **carotid body**. It serves as chemical sensing center for blood gases (e.g., blood gases during exercise such as O2, CO2), which communicates action potentials (electrical messages) to the CNS via the **glossopharyngeal nerve** (CN IX). This triggers the respiratory center of the brain to change respiration rate and attempts to restore homeostasis of blood gases. Similar to the carotid body, the **carotid sinus** is an expansion of the internal carotid wall at the most proximal location. Specialized mechanical receptors, called **baroreceptors**, in the arterial wall sense changes in blood pressure (e.g.,

Figure 4-1

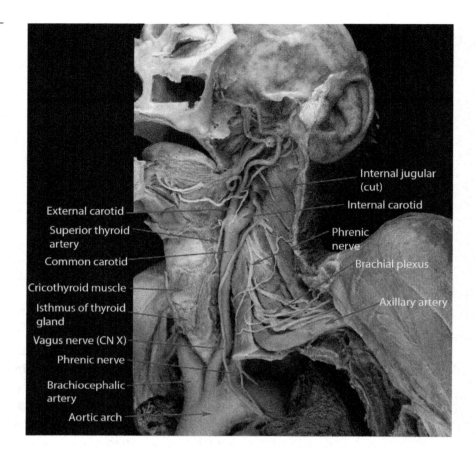

Internal jugular (cut)

Internal carotid

External carotid

Superior thyroid artery

Common carotid

Phrenic nerve

Cricothyroid muscle

Brachial plexus

Isthmus of thyroid gland

Axillary artery

Vagus nerve (CN X)

Phrenic nerve

Brachiocephalic artery

Aortic arch

supine position to standing). The glossopharyngeal nerve (CN IX) communicates sensory action potentials to the CNS helping to restore homoeostatic blood pressure by altering heart rate and cardiac output.

What is the cardiovascular response to standing and the baroreceptor reflex? What is orthostatic hypotension?

The cardiovascular response to standing from a supine position includes the pull of blood inferiorly and venous pooling in the lower limb. Blood from the lower body must now return to the heart against the pull of gravity. The resulting physiologic response is baroreceptor stimulation within the carotid sinus and increased glossopharyngeal nerve (CN IX) activity. The CNS receives the electrical messages from CN IX and responds by increasing cardiac output. However, a prolonged decrease (several minutes) in mean arterial blood pressure and less perfusion to the brain (i.e., light headedness) in this setting is called **orthostatic hypotension**. The etiology of this condition is not clear, but risk factors include aging, dehydration, nutrition, autonomic failure, Parkinson's disease, spinal cord injury, and CNS lesions (Robertson, 2008).

What are the internal jugular, external jugular, and anterior jugular veins?

The **internal jugular vein** is located deep to the sternocleidomastoid muscle within the carotid sheath **(see figure 4-2)**.

Figure 4-2

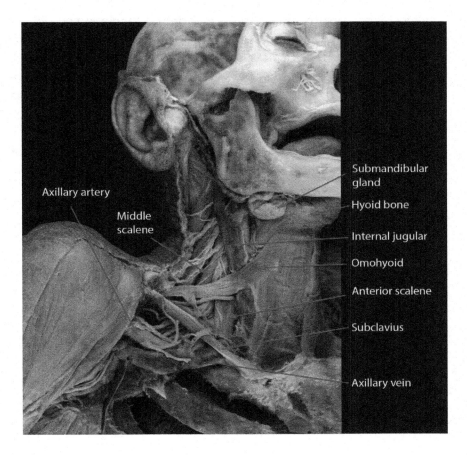

Axillary artery

Middle scalene

Submandibular gland

Hyoid bone

Internal jugular

Omohyoid

Anterior scalene

Subclavius

Axillary vein

Blood drains from the brain to the internal jugular through the **jugular foramen** in the skull. It then drains into the brachiocephalic vein. The **external jugular vein** receives blood from the scalp, facial region, and anterior neck, and drains into the proximal subclavian vein. It courses over the superficial aspect of the sternocleidomastoid muscle in the neck. The **anterior jugular vein** drains the superficial anterior neck into the external jugular.

How is the neck compartmentalized?

Similar to the upper and lower limbs, the neck is compartmentalized via deep cervical fascia. The fascia can limit the spread of infection and hemorrhaging (blood loss) in this region. However, the thorax and head regions are accessible within each defined compartment. The **investing layer** is the most superficial layer of deep investing fascia that surrounds the circumference of the neck. This layer envelopes the trapezius and sternocleidomastoid muscles. The **pre-vertebral fascia** is beneath the deep investing fascia. It surrounds the vertebral column and most skeletal muscles in the deep neck (erector spinae, transversospinalis, and scalenes). The **pretracheal fascia** in the anterior neck surrounds the trachea, esophagus, thyroid gland, and parathyroid gland. The **buccopharyngeal fascia** is a component of the pre-tracheal fascia located on its posterior aspect. The bilateral **carotid sheath,** located anterolaterally, surrounds the carotid artery, internal jugular vein, vagus nerve (CN X), and lymph nodes. The **alar fascia** lies between the two carotid sheaths and the **retropharyngeal space** is lies between this and the pre-vertebral fascia.

See CM 4-1A, 4-1B, and 4-1C for Review.

CM 4-1A

Vasculature and Fascia

↓

Arterial

↓

Delivers arterial blood
to brain, face, scalp

↓

Common carotid

Located at
the bifurcation
of common
carotid; specialized
chemoreceptor
cells for sensing
blood gases

↓

Carotid body

to brain; courses
deep and enters
carotid opening of skull

To face, scrap;
courses behind
mandible

→ **External carotid**

↓

Internal carotid

↓

expansion of proximal internal carotid;
machanical receptors to sense arterial
wall stretch (baroreceptor)

↓

Orthostatic hypotension — *Impaired ability to improve blood pressure upon standing* — **Carotid sinus**

↓

relays sensory
input to CNS

↓

Glossopharyngeal nerve (CN IX)

CM 4-1B

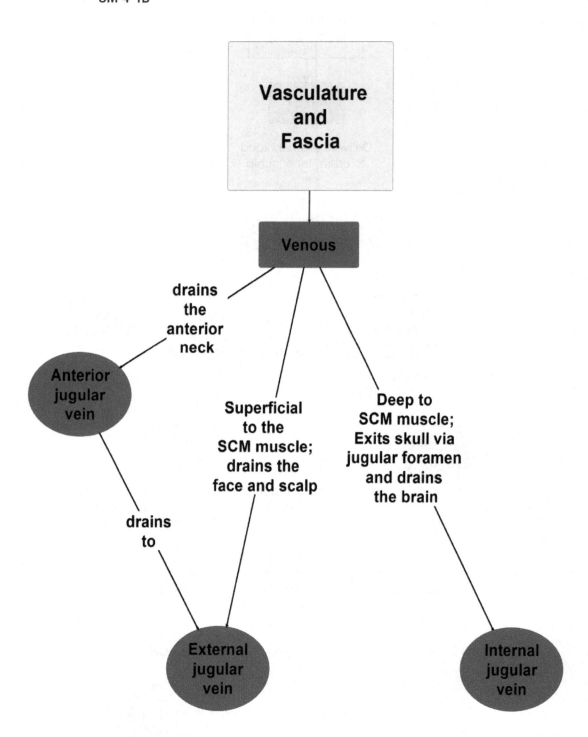

CM 4-1C

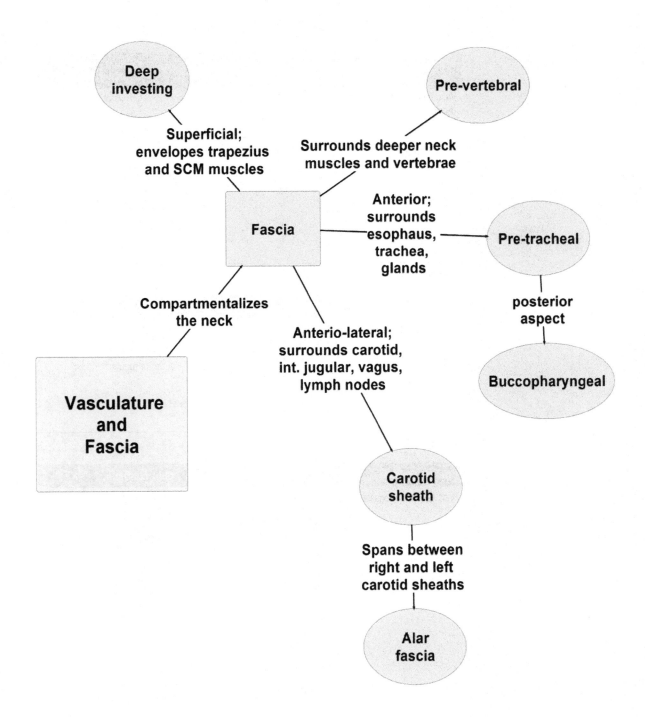

Synthesis Exercise: Create a concept map using items from EXERCISE 4-1A, 4-1B, and 4-1C.

Exercise 4-1A

Primary Category	Secondary Category	Continuations	Clinical Considerations
Vasculature and fascia	Arterial	Common carotid	Orthostatic hypotension
		Internal carotid	
		External carotid	
		Carotid sinus	
		Carotid body	
		Glossopharyngeal nerve (CN IX)	

Exercise 4-1B

Primary Category	Secondary Category	Continuations
Vasculature and fascia	Venous	Internal jugular
		External jugular
		Anterior jugular

Exercise 4-1C

Primary Category	Secondary Category	Continuations
Vasculature and fascia	Fascia	Deep investing
		Pre-vertebral
		Pre-tracheal
		Carotid sheath
		Alar fascia
		Buccopharyngeal fascia

II. Superficial Neck (anterior and lateral)

Overview of key topics for this section:

- Platysma muscle
- Sternocleidomastoid muscle and triangles of the neck
- Nerve point and cutaneous innervation of the neck
- Submandibular gland
- Hyoid bone
- Suprahyoid muscles
- Infrahyoid muscles
- Ansa Cervicalis and the cervical plexus

What is the platysma muscle?

The **platysma muscle** is located very superficially in the neck and helps enable facial expression. It attaches from the mandibular region (lower lip, angle of mouth, cheek) to the clavicular region. Innervation is via the cervical branch of facial nerve (CN VII).

What is the sternocleidomastoid muscle? What are the borders of the lateral triangle of the neck (posterior triangle)? Anterior cervical region of the neck (anterior triangle)? Where is the posterior triangle of the neck?

The **stenocleidomastoid (SCM) muscle** is a key landmark within the neck region **(see figure 4-3)**.

The SCM attaches from the mastoid process of the temporal bone, to the medial clavicle (clavicular head) and the manubrium of the sternum (sternal head). Unilateral contraction promotes cervical rotation to the opposite side and bilateral contraction flexes the neck. The spinal accessory nerve (CN XI) innervates the SCM. The SCM constitutes the sternocleidomastoid region, which separates the anterior and lateral cervical regions.

The anterior border of the trapezius and the posterior border of the SCM create the **lateral cervical region (posterior triangle)**. The union of the

Figure 4-3

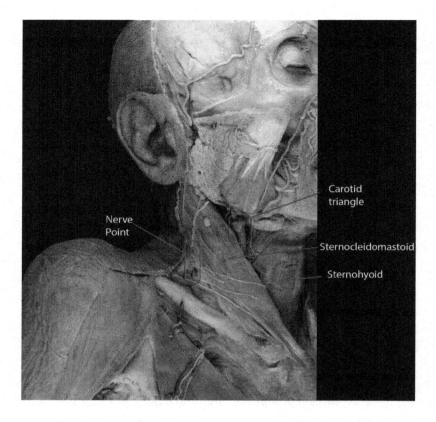

Carotid triangle

Nerve Point

Sternocleidomastoid

Sternohyoid

SCM and trapezius form the boundary of the apex and the middle third of the clavicle forms the inferior border. The lateral cervical region contains muscles (scalenes, levator scapulae, splenius, and omohyoid), vasculature (subclavian artery, transverse cervical artery, and suprascapular artery), nerves (spinal accessory, branches of cervical plexus, and roots and trunks of the brachial plexus), and lymph nodes.

The anterior border of SCM and midline of the anterior neck establish the **anterior cervical region (anterior triangle)**. The lower border of the mandible forms the superior boundary, and the jugular notch of the manubrium of the sternum forms an inferior boundary. Within the anterior cervical region are suprahyoid and infrahyoid muscles, which are named for their location relative to the hyoid bone. Also, the infrahyoid and suprahyoid muscles create a subdivision called the **carotid triangle.** Another subdivision**, the submandibular (digastric) triangle,** is located between the lower border of the mandible and the suprahyoid. Similarly**, the submental triangle** is found just inferior to the anterior aspect of the mandibular symphysis.

Created by the trapezius muscle, the **posterior cervical region** is a distinct region from the lateral cervical region (posterior triangle).

What is the nerve point? What provides cutaneous innervation to the neck?

Just posterior to the SCM muscle four cutaneous nerves exit at the **nerve point** of the neck(**see figure 4-3**). The cervical plexus is the origin of these nerves, which include the following: (1) **supraclavicular nerve** (innervatesnear the clavicle and above), (2) **transverse cervical nerve** (innervates the anterior neck), (3) **lesser occipital nerve** (innervates posterior to the auricle of the ear and the lateral occipital region), and (4) **great auricular nerve** (innervates the auricle of ear and anterior to the auricle). Dorsal rami from cervical spinal nerves help innervate the skin of the posterior neck.

Where is the submandibular gland and its basic function?

The **submandibular gland** is located superior to the digastric muscle and inferior to the mandible and a portion is found deep to the mandible. It secretes saliva into the oral cavity via the submandibular duct with increased parasympathetic activity. The chorda tympani of the facial nerve (CN VII) provide parasympathetic innervation to the submandibular gland (more detail in Chapter 8: Head).

What are the suprahyoid muscles, their attachments, and their functions?

The **suprahyoid muscles** are located superior to the hyoid bone **(see figure 4-4)**.

This group of muscles include the (1) **digastric** (anterior and posterior belly, which attaches from the mandible to the hyoid bone to the mastoid process), (2) **geniohyoid** (attaches from the mandibular symphysis to the hyoid bone), (3) **stylohyoid** (attaches from the styloid process to the hyoid bone), and (4) **mylohyoid** (attaches from the mylohyoid line of the mandible to the hyoid bone). Taken together, the suprahyoid muscles function to elevate the hyoid bone, which is necessary to propel a food bolus into the pharynx.

Figure 4-4

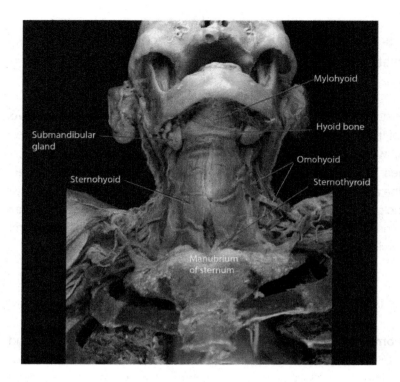

Mylohyoid

Hyoid bone

Submandibular gland

Omohyoid

Sternothyroid

Sternohyoid

Manubrium of sternum

What are the infrahyoid muscles their attachments, functions, and innervation?

Lying inferior to the hyoid bone **(see figure 4-4),** the **infrahyoid muscles** include (1) **sternohyoid** (attaches from the **manubrium** of sternum to the hyoid bone), (2) **omohyoid** (attaches from the scapula to the medial clavicle to the hyoid), (3) **thyrohyoid** (attaches from the thyroid cartilage to the hyoid bone), and (4) **sternothyroid** (attaches from the manubrium of the sternum to the thyroid cartilage. Only the C1 spinal nerve innervates the thyrohyoid, while the ansa cervicalis (C1–C3) innervated the remaining three muscles in this group.

What is the ansa cervicalis?

The **ansa cervicalis** is a loop of motor nerves, which reside near the bifurcation of the common carotid artery and receives branches from the cervical plexus (C1–C3). The **superior loop** of the ansa cervicalis receives a branch from C1 and the **inferior loop** from C2–C3. Taken together, the motor nerves innervate three of the four infrahyoid muscles (the sterno-hyoid, sternothyroid, and omohyoid). However, the thyrohyoid muscle is innervated only by C1, not the ansa cervicalis.

See CM 4-2A and 4-2B for Review.

CM 4-2A

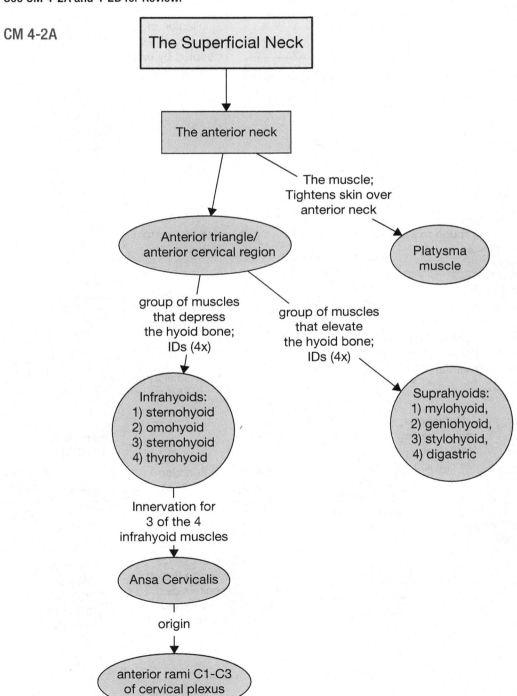

CM 4-2B

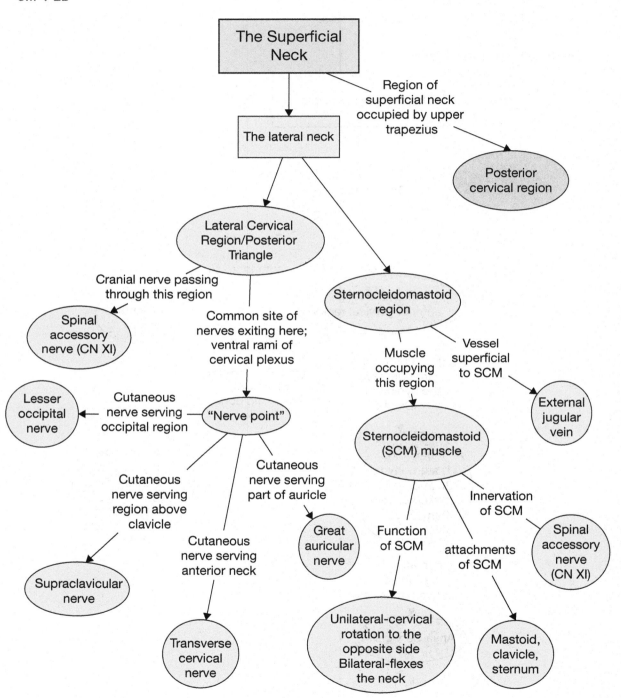

Synthesis Exercise: Create a concept map using items from EXERCISE 4-2A and 4-2B.

Exercise 4-2A

Primary Category	Secondary Category	Continuations
The superficial neck	The anterior neck	Platysma muscle
		Anterior triangle / anterior cervical region
		Infrahyoid
		Sternohyoid
		Omohyoid
		Sternohyoid
		Thyrohyoid
		Suprahyoid
		Mylohyoid
		Geniohyoid
		Stylohyoid
		Digastric
		Ansa Cervicalis
		Anterior rami C1-C3 of cervical plexus

Exercise 4-2B

Primary Category	Secondary Category	Continuations
The superficial neck	The lateral neck	Lateral cervical region / posterior triangle
	Posterior cervical region	Sternocleidomastoid region
		"Nerve point"
		Lesser occipital nerve
		Supraclavicular nerve
		Transverse cervical nerve
		Great auricular nerve
		External jugular vein
		Spinal accessory nerve (CN XI)
		Mastoid
		Clavicle
		Sternum
		Unilateral- cervical rotation to the opposite side Bilateral- flexes the neck

III. Deep Neck (larynx, glands, *and Other Features*)

Overview of key topics for this section:

- Hyoid bone
- Thyroid gland
- Pyramidal, or accessory lobe, of thyroid gland
- Thyroglossal duct cyst
- Parathyroid gland
- Plasma calcium regulation
- Larynx and laryngeal cartilage
- Tracheostomy
- Laryngeal nerves (superior, inferior)
- Laryngeal muscles
- Vocal cords, vocal folds, voice production, and pitch
- Laryngitis
- Superior deep cervical lymph nodes

Where is the hyoid bone located? What is its shape and its function? Why is this bone studied in forensic medicine?

The **hyoid bone** is a horseshoe, or U-shaped bone located anteriorly within the neck. It resides at approximately the C3 vertebrae level between the mandible and thyroid cartilage. Major features of the hyoid bone include the **greater horns**, **lesser horns**, and **body**. The suprahyoid and infrahyoid muscles attach to the hyoid bone to facilitate its movement during swallowing. During forensic investigations, a fractured hyoid bone can indicate strangulation as a cause of death.

What are the scalene muscles? What are the pre-vertebral muscles?

The **scalene muscles** (anterior, middle, and posterior) reside bilaterally in the deep neck (**see figure 4-2**). They attach from cervical vertebrae C2–C7 to the first and second ribs to elevate the same ribs. The **prevertebral muscles** of the deep neck include the (1) **longus capitus** (flexes at the atlanto-occipital joint), (2) **longus colli** (flexes head and neck), 3) **rectus capitus anterior** (flexes at the atlanto-occipital joint), and (4) **rectus capitus lateralis** (lateral flexion, stability of atlanto-occipital joint).

Where is the thyroid gland located? What is its shape and its function?

The **thyroid gland** lies anterolateral to the superior cartilaginous rings of the trachea (**see figure 4-1**). It has two lobes (right, left). A midline portion of the gland, called the **isthmus**, connects the lobes. The thyroid gland is activated by thyroid stimulating hormone from the anterior pituitary gland. In response it secretes **thyroid hormones (T3, T4)** which regulate growth and energy production of the body. The thyroid gland receives blood supply from the **superior thyroid artery** (branches of the external carotid) and **inferior thyroid arteries** (branch of the thyrocervical trunk).

What is a pyramidal or accessory lobe of the thyroid gland? A thyroglossal duct cyst?

The thyroid gland begins near the posterior aspect of the tongue and tracks inferiorly to its final location in the neck. A **pyramidal,** or **accessory lobe** of thyroid gland, located midline and superior to the gland may persist following the development of the thyroid gland. midline=Also, a **thyroglossal duct** or **canal** can persist following development and tracking of the thyroid gland. However, it frequently atrophies and does not remain patent (open). In some cases, the duct remains patent and can potentially facilitate a bacterial infection, called a **thyroglossal duct cyst**.

Where are the parathyroid glands located? What are their function? What are aberrant parathyroid glands?

The four **parathyroid glands** are typically located on the posterior surface of thyroid gland, with two on each side. Following a decrease in blood calcium levels, they secrete **parathyroid hormone** (PTH) into the blood to increase calcium reabsorption from the digestive tract and bone. Once blood calcium homeostasis is restored, PTH secretion is reduced. Aberrant parathyroid glands can exist both above and below the thyroid cartilage.

Where is the larynx located? What provides structural support of the larynx?

The **larynx** (or voice box) is found at the C3–C6 vertebral level near the anterior neck and connects the inferior aspect of the pharynx with the trachea. Paired and unpaired cartilage form the laryngeal skeleton, providing structural support for the larynx. Paired cartilage includes the **arytenoid**, which creates tension or slack in vocal cords to change pitch of voice, **corniculate,** a horn-shaped cartilage at the apex of the arytenoid), and **cuneiform**, which are club-shaped cartilage, anterior to the corniculate. Unpaired cartilage of the larynx comprises the **epiglottis** (a heart-shaped superior lid), **thyroid cartilage** (largest cartilage with laryngeal prominence), and **cricoid cartilage** (ring shaped and inferior to thyroid cartilage). The **median cricothyroid ligament** spans the cricoid and thyroid cartilage in the midline of the neck. A **thyrohyoid membrane** spans thyroid cartilage and hyoid bone and serves as a site of entry for the internal branch of the superior laryngeal artery and nerve.

What is a tracheostomy?

Patients with an upper respiratory obstruction or respiratory failure may require a tracheostomy. During this emergency procedure, a medical practitioner makes a small incision between the upper cartilaginous rings of the trachea, and inserts of a tracheostomy tube into the airway. Several important blood vessels are present in this region, such as the inferior thyroid veins, the thyroid ima artery, and the left brachiocephalic vein.

What is the mechanism for voice production? What is the mechanism for increasing and decreasing the pitch of the voice?

Vibrations of the true vocal cords produce the voice, facilitated by the outward flow of the air of respiration. The **vocal ligaments** (or true vocal cords), made of elastic tissue, are attached from the arytenoid cartilage to the thyroid cartilage, and are covered by a mucosal membrane called the **vocal fold**. The length of the vocal cords and the frequency of vibrations determine the pitch of audible sound. For example, elongated or stretched vocal cords produce a higher frequency of vibration and higher pitch. Conversely, relaxed or shortened vocal cords result in a lower frequency of vibration and lower pitch. A simple analogy is comparing the actions of the vocal cords to the vibrations made by a rubber band. A variety of muscles (listed below) promote lengthening and shortening of the vocal cords to change pitch. In contrast, the **vestibular ligaments** (or false vocal cords) do not contribute to voice production. They are enveloped by a mucosal membrane and and the combined structure is known as the **vestibular fold**. Males tend to possess lower pitched voices due to their longer vocal cords, compared to those of females. This structural feature is supported by the increased production of testosterone in males. In addition to altering length, the vocal cords can also change their location. The aperture or space between the vocal folds, called the **rima glottis** can be closed during adduction, or opened during abduction of the vocal cords.

What muscles act on the larynx? What innervates the muscles of the larynx? What innervates the mucosa of the larynx?

Several muscles influence the length and location of vocal cords in the larynx. They are listed below with their respective function. Note: the cricothyroid muscle is the single muscle located superficially and outside of the larynx. It receives different innervation than the muscles located deeply and posterior in the larynx.

Vocal Cord Muscles

1. Cricothyroid muscles: lengthen and stretch the vocal folds, increasing pitch

2. Thyroarytenoid muscles: relaxes vocal chords

3. Posterior cricoarytenoid muscles: abduct vocal folds

4. Lateral cricoarytenoid muscles: adduct vocal folds

5. Transverse arytenoid muscle: adduct vocal folds

6. Oblique arytenoid muscles: adduct and narrow the **laryngeal inlet**

7. **Vocalis muscles**: relax the posterior aspect of the vocal ligaments

Motor innervation to the muscles of the larynx relies on the **recurrent laryngeal nerve** (a branch from the vagus nerve; CN X), except for the cricothyroid muscle, which innervated by the **external branch of the superior laryngeal nerve** (a branch from the vagus nerve; CN X). Sensory innervation to the larynx above the vocal folds is via the **internal branch of superior laryngeal nerve**. However, the recurrent laryngeal nerve innervates the mucosa of the larynx below the vocal folds. The vocal folds specifically receive sensory innervation from both the internal branch of the superior laryngeal nerve and the recurrent laryngeal nerve.

What is laryngitis?

Laryngitis is inflammation and swelling of the vocal chords. Depending on the stimulus, it can persist for a few days (acute) or several weeks (chronic). Some causes include overuse (e.g., excessive yelling), bacterial or viral infection, and acid reflux disease. A patient with laryngitis may experience weak voice production and discomfort within the larynx.

Where are the superior deep cervical lymph nodes? What is the significance of palpating these lymph nodes?

The majority of lymph fluid from the superficial neck, face, and head drains into the superior cervical lymph nodes, found bilaterally near the angle of mandible. Lymph fluid subsequently drains to the inferior cervical lymph nodes. Palpating the superior cervical lymph nodes allows clinicians to check for enlargement during a bacterial or viral infection.

See CM 4-3A and 4-3B for Review.

CM 4-3A

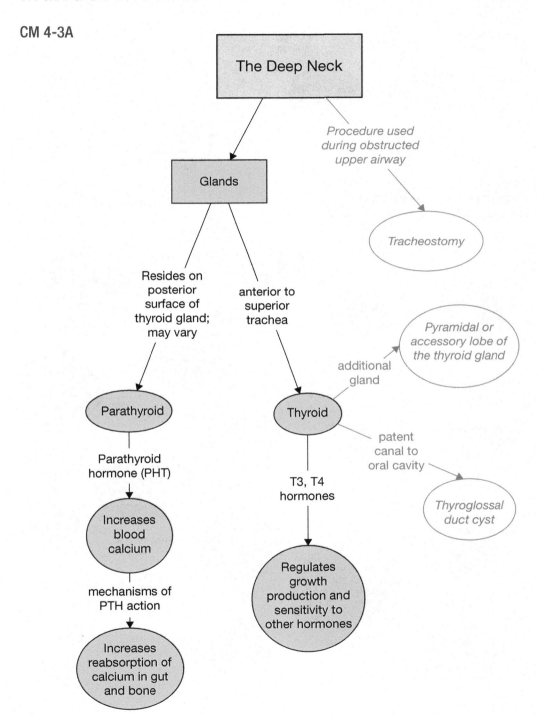

CM 4-3B

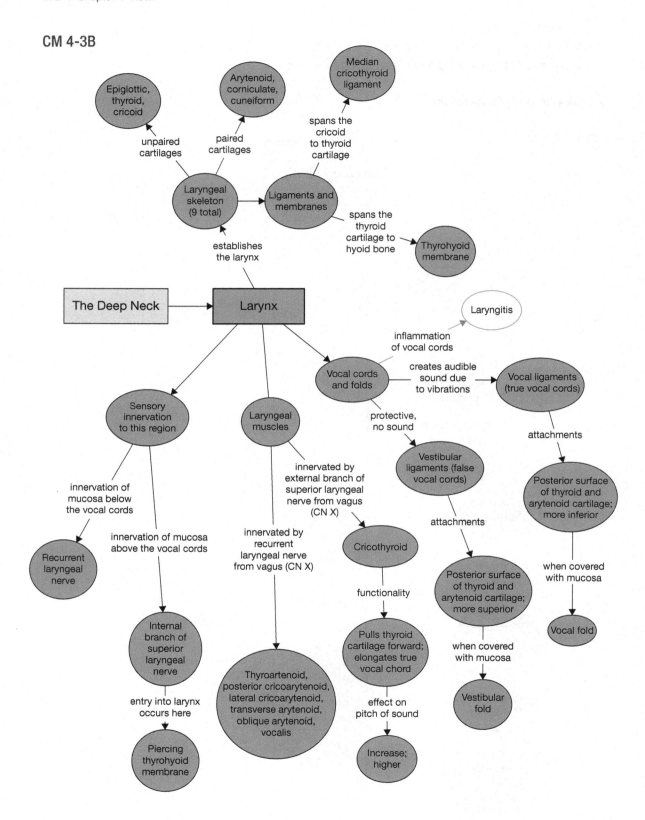

Synthesis Exercise: Create a concept map using items from EXERCISE 4-3A and 4-3B.

Exercise 4-3A

Primary Category	Secondary Category	Continuations	Clinical Considerations
The deep neck	Glands	Thyroid Parathyroid Regulates growth and sensitivity to other hormones Increases blood calcium Increases reabsorption of calcium in gut and bone	Tracheostomy Pyramidal or accessory lobe of thyroid Thyroglossal duct cyst

Exercise 4-3B

Primary Category	Secondary Categories	Continuations	Clinical Considerations
The deep neck	Larynx	Laryngeal skeleton (9 total) Ligaments and membranes Vocal cords and folds Laryngeal Muscles Sensory innervation to larynx Thyroid Epiglottic Cricoid Arytenoid Corniculate Cuneiform Median cricothyroid ligament Thyrohyoid membrane Vocal ligaments (true vocal cords) Vestibular ligaments (false vocal cords) Cricothyroid muscle Thyroartenoid muscle posterior cricoarytenoid muscle lateral cricoarytenoid muscle	Laryngitis

Primary Category	Secondary Categories	Continuations	Clinical Considerations
		transverse arytenoid muscle	
		oblique arytenoid muscle	
		Vocalis muscle	
		Internal branch of superior laryngeal nerve	
		Recurrent laryngeal nerve	
		Posterior surface of thyroid and arytenoid cartilage	
		Posterior surface of thyroid and arytenoid cartilage	
		pulls thyroid cartilage forward; elongates vocal chord	
		Vocal fold	
		Vestibular fold	
		Increase; higher	
		Piercing thyrohyoid membrane	
		Vocalis muscle	
		Internal branch of superior laryngeal nerve	
		Recurrent laryngeal nerve	
		Posterior surface of thyroid and arytenoid cartilage	
		Posterior surface of thyroid and arytenoid cartilage	
		pulls thyroid cartilage forward; elongates vocal chord	
		Vocal fold	
		Vestibular fold	
		Increase; higher	
		Piercing thyrohyoid membrane	

Image Credits

- Fig. 4-1: Copyright © 2016 by 4D Anatomy. Reprinted with permission.
- Fig. 4-2: Copyright © 2016 by 4D Anatomy. Reprinted with permission.
- Fig. 4-3: Copyright © 2016 by 4D Anatomy. Reprinted with permission.
- Fig. 4-4: Copyright © 2016 by 4D Anatomy. Reprinted with permission.

Chapter 5

Head

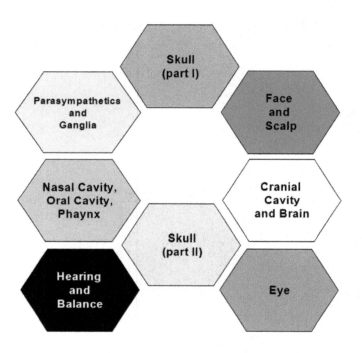

Brief Overview

What anatomic features are included?

The head is the most superior region in the anatomical position and serves as an entry point for a variety of special sensory functions, such as vision, hearing, taste, balance, and olfaction (smell). The brain is housed within the bony skull for protection. Twelve cranial nerves (CN I–XII) exit the skull through foramina or hollow passageways. As previously discussed in Chapter 1, cranial nerves can have functions related to motor processing, sensory processing, or both. In this chapter, the head will be subdivided into eight specific topics (**see figure 5-1**). Cranial nerve target tissue and functionality will be explained as we proceed through these topics.

I. Skull — Part I

Overview of key topics for this section:

- Plates of the skull (neurocranium)
- Facial bones and mandible (viscerocranium)
- Temporomandibular joint

What are the major plates of the skull? What are the sites of articulation between each plate?

The region of skull that surrounds and protects the brain is called the **neurocranium**. Several plate-like bones articulate together to form sutures or sutural joints. The single **frontal bone** is located superiorly and anteriorly and is often referred to as the *forehead*. The bilateral **parietal bones** are posterior to the frontal bone. The frontal and parietal bones articulate through the **coronal suture** and are within the coronal plane. The right and left parietal bones articulate via the **sagittal suture** which is located in the sagittal plane. The coronal and sagittal sutures intersect at a location called the **bregma**. A single **occipital bone** is found posterior and inferior to the parietal bones. It includes a surface anatomy landmark called the **external occipital protuberance** and articulates with both the parietal and the temporal bones. The location where a prominent sutural line located between the occipital and parietal bones, called the **lambdoid suture**, intersects with the sagittal suture is referred to as the **lambda,** for its resemblance to the lower case Greek letter. The bilateral **temporal bones,** located at the base of the lateral walls of the cranium has several unique features such as the **mastoid process**, the **styloid process**, the **external acoustic meatus** (or ear canal), and **zygomatic process** of the zygomatic arch, which forms part of the cheek bone. The **temporal fossa** and **infratemporal fossa** lie just superior and inferior to the zygomatic arch, respectively. The **sphenoid bone,** found inferior to the frontal bone, primarily resides deeper inside the skull. It possesses a **central body, greater wings** (right and left), and **lesser wings** (right and left). The intersection of four skull plates, called the **pterion**, is located between the frontal, parietal, sphenoid, and temporal bones. It is a relatively weak site of the bony skull and susceptible to fracture (e.g., impact with baseball or fist). The inferior and deep aspects of the skull will be discussed in Skull — Part II.

What are the facial bones of the skull? What is the mandible?

The **viscerocranium** (or facial skeleton) is an anteriorly located portion of the skull comprised of irregularly shaped facial bones and the mandible. It serves to protect a portion of the orbital socket, nasal cavity, and oral cavity. The **nasal bone** (bridge of the nose) is centrally located and articulates with the inferior aspect of the frontal bone via the **nasion**. Inferior to the nasal bone is the maxillary bone. It possesses a central hollow region, called the **nasal cavity**, which is divided by the **vomer** and perpendicular plate of the deep **ethmoid bone**. Together, these bones create a **nasal septum,** which separates the right versus the left nasal cavities. The maxillary bone houses the upper row of teeth (or maxillary teeth) through **alveolar processes**, or sockets for the roots of the teeth. It also contributes to the medial and inferior aspect of the orbit. The **lacrimal bone**, which houses the lacrimal sac, can be found just posterior to the upper maxillary bone. An **infraorbital foramen** allows the infraorbital nerve and artery to reach the surface of the mid-face from within the maxillary bone. The paired **zygomatic bone** (or cheek bone) is found lateral to the maxillary bone. It also contributes to the zygomatic arch as well as a portion of the lateral orbit.

The mandible forms the lower aspect of the facial region and oral cavity. It houses the lower row of teeth (or mandibular teeth) via alveolar processes. The horizontal **body of the mandible** projects anteriorly while the **ramus of the mandible** is aligned in the vertical direction and the site where they meet is called the **angle of the mandible**. On the superior and posterior aspects, the **condyle** includes the head and neck of the mandible. The **coronoid process** projects anteriorly, relative to the condyle. The **mandibular notch** separates these superior projections. A bilateral **mental foramen** on the anterior and center aspects of the mandible allows the mental nerve to exit the inferior face via the mandible. The **mandibular foramen** on the medial and posterior aspects permits the inferior alveolar nerve and artery to enter the deep bone. This nerve is responsible for innervation to all of the mandibular teeth; the distal branches are commonly anesthetized by a dentist.

What is the temporomandibular joint?

The **temporomandibular joint** (or TMJ) is an articulation site between the head of the mandibular condyle and the mandibular fossa of the temporal bone. It allows the mandible to open and close during speech and mastication of food. Parts of the TMJ include a synovial membrane, an articular disc, and a joint capsule. This joint may experience arthritis due to a variety of factors such as infections, trauma, and aging. It may also become dislocated if the head of the mandible excessively translates in the anterior direction.

See CM 5-1A and 5-1B for Review.

CM 5-1A

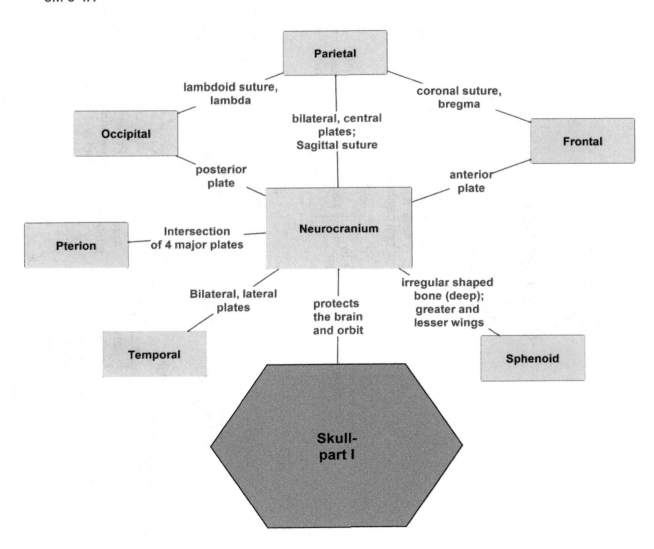

CM 5-1B

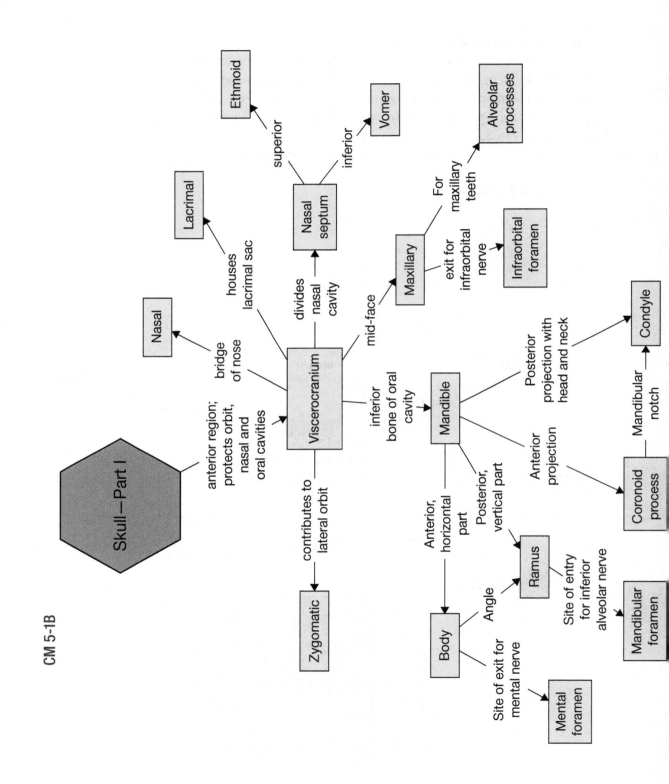

Synthesis Exercise: Create a concept map using items from EXERCISE 5-1A and 5-1B.

Exercise 5-1A

Primary Category	Secondary Category	Continuations
Skull — Part I	Neurocranium	Frontal
		Parietal
		Occipital
		Temporal
		Sphenoid
		Pterion

Exercise 5-1B

Primary Category	Secondary Category	Continuations
Skull — Part I	Viscerocranium	Nasal
		Lacrimal
		Nasal septum
		Ethmoid
		Vomer
		Maxillary
		Mandible
		Zygomatic
		Alveolar processes
		Infraorbital foramen
		Body
		Ramus
		Condyle
		Coronoid process
		Mandibular foramen
		Mental foramen

II. Face and Scalp

Overview of key topics for this section:

- Muscles of facial expression
- Facial nerve
- Bell's Palsy
- Chorda tympani branch
- Arterial supply to the superficial face, tongue, deep face, and scalp
- Venous drainage of the face and scalp
- Parotid gland
- Layers of the scalp
- Trigeminal nerve (CN V)

What are the muscles of facial expression?

The facial region includes a variety of unique skeletal muscles that promote facial expression (e.g., surprised), protect the eyes, enable speech, and assist with mastication of food **(see figures 5-1, 5-2, 5-3).** Superficial to the frontal bone of the skull is the **frontal belly of the occipitofrontalis muscle**. It can raise and wrinkle the skin over the frontal bone (forehead) when a person is surprised. The **orbicularis oculi muscle** surrounds the orbit in two parts and functions to close the surrounding skin over the eyeball. The general shape of the muscle is circular. An **orbital part** is located around the circumference of the orbit and promotes a sphincter-like action of the skin (e.g., like an expression you might make in a dust storm). The **palpebral part** overlays the central aspect of the orbit (the eyelids) and helps close the eye during typical daily function (e.g., blinking). The **levator labi superioris** attaches to the medial upper labia (lip) elevating the labia. **Levator anguli oris** is located more laterally and raises the corners of the mouth. **Zygomaticus minor** (smaller, medial) and **zygomaticus major** (larger, lateral) help to elevate the corners of mouth. A **risorius** muscle also assists in smiling. Similar to the orbicularis oculi of the orbit, the **orbicularis oris** is a circular shaped muscle surrounding the mouth, which closes of the mouth, much like a sphincter (e.g., drinking from a straw, kissing, speaking.

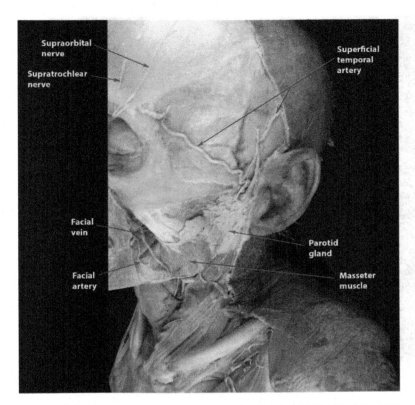

Figure 5-1

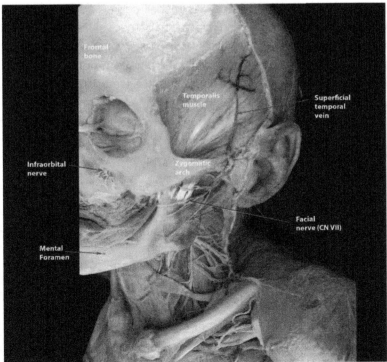

Figure 5-2

Figure 5-3

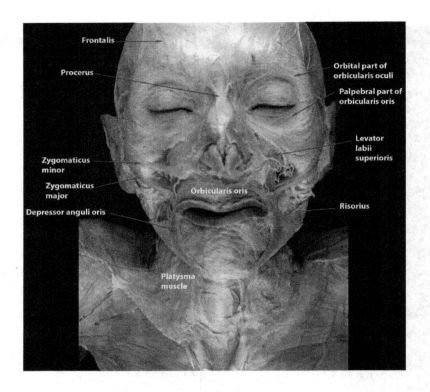

Frontalis

Procerus

Orbital part of
orbicularis oculi

Palpebral part of
orbicularis oris

Levator
labii
superioris

Zygomaticus
minor

Zygomaticus
major

Orbicularis oris

Depressor anguli oris

Risorius

Platysma
muscle

whistling). The **depressor labi inferioris** (medial) depresses the lower lip and the **depressor anguli oris** (lateral) draws the corners of the mouth inferior. Located in a plane deep to the masseter muscle and within the buccal fat pad of the cheek is the **buccinator,** which helps propel food from the buccal pocket of the oral cavity (or cheek) into the teeth for continued mastication. The **mentalis** muscle, located inferior to the lower labia, protrudes the lower labia when contracted (e.g., pouting face). A very thin muscle called the **platysma** spans the anterior neck and attaches superiorly on the lower mandible. It helps tighten the skin over the neck and also assists in depression of the lower labia (e.g., surprised or horrified).

What is the facial nerve (CN VII)? What are the superficial branches and respective functions?

The facial nerve (CN VII) provides six major branches: five to the superficial face and one to the occipital region **(see figure 5-2)**. It exits the skull from the stylomastoid foramen (more on this structure in Skull — Part II) and five of the six distal branches course through the parotid gland as the parotid plexus. All six distal branches of CN VII are listed below with the associated motor innervation to the respective muscles (e.g., nerve branch → muscles innervated).

Facial Nerves

1. temporal branch: frontal belly of occipitofrontalis, superior aspect of orbicularis oculi

2. zygomatic branch: inferior aspect of orbicular oculi, zygomaticus major and minor

3. buccal branch: buccinator, superior labial muscles

4. marginal mandibular branch: inferior labial muscles

5. cervical branch: platysma muscle

✓ *A common learning mnemonic to recall the distal branches of CN VII to the anterior face is:* **T**en **Z**ebras **B**it **M**y **C**heek

6. posterior auricular branch: occipital belly of occipitofrontalis muscle

What is Bell's palsy?

Bell's palsy paralyzes he facial muscles unilaterally. One half of the face remains dormant on the ipsilateral side while the contralateral side is unaffected. For example, a patient can exhibit smiling on the unaffected side. Causes of Bell's palsy include herpes zoster virus infection, trauma, stroke, and surgical lesion of the facial nerve.

What is the chorda tympani? What it its function?

The **chorda tympani** is a branch from the facial nerve (CNVII) that relays special sensory tastes (e.g., bitter, sweet, sour) from the anterior two thirds of the tongue. The lingual nerve of trigeminal nerve (CN V3) conveys fibers from the chorda tympani.

What arteries supply the tongue, superficial face, deep face, and scalp?

A primary arterial supply to the tongue, superficial face, deep face, and scalp is the external carotid artery. The **lingual artery** branches proximally and anteriorly from the external carotid to supply the tongue. Also branching from the anterior aspect of the external carotid is the **facial artery,** which courses over the middle body of the mandible to supply the superficial face **(see figure 5-1)**. It provides **superior and inferior labial arteries** to the oral region. The facial artery continues towards the nasal cartilage as the **lateral nasal artery** and **angular artery**. Other branches stem from the external carotid artery, such as the **occipital artery** (occipital region of the skull), the **posterior auricular artery** (posterior to the auricle, or ear) and the **maxillary artery** (primarily to the deeper face) **(see figure 5-4)**. Several specific branches arise from the maxillary artery, such as the **inferior alveolar artery** (to the mandible and lower teeth), the **masseteric** and **pterygoid branches** (to the masseter and pterygoid muscles), **middle meningeal artery** (to dura mater and skull), **deep temporal arteries** (to the temporalis muscle), the **buccal artery** (to the buccal region, or cheek), the **descending palatine artery** (to the palate), the **sphenopalatine artery** (to the nasal cavity), the **posterior superior alveolar artery** (to the maxilla and upper row of teeth), and the **infraorbital artery**

Figure 5-4

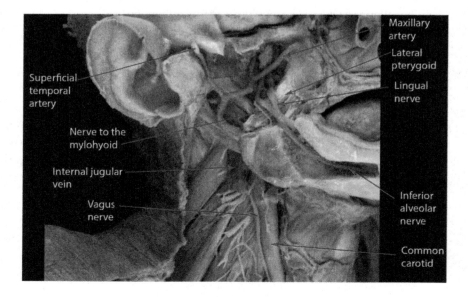

Superficial temporal artery

Nerve to the mylohyoid

Internal jugular vein

Vagus nerve

Maxillary artery

Lateral pterygoid

Lingual nerve

Inferior alveolar nerve

Common carotid

(to the mid-superficial face). As a direct superior continuation of the external artery, the **superficial temporal artery** helps supply the anastomosis of the scalp **(see figure 5-1)**. This extensive network of arteries provides a rich blood supply to the scalp and contributes to extensive blood loss, or hemorrhaging, following a scalp laceration. However, some of the arterial supply to this anastomosis originates from the internal carotid artery and not the external carotid. For example, the two bilateral **supratrochlear** and two **supraorbital** arteries exit the skull near the superior-medial aspect of the orbit to supply the scalp with blood. The origin of these blood vessels is the **ophthalmic artery** (to the eyeball) from the internal carotid artery. Taken together, five arteries (occipital, posterior auricular, superficial temporal, supratrochlear, and supraorbital) anastomose and contribute blood to the scalp.

How is venous blood drained from the face and scalp?

Venous drainage from the face and scalp includes several vessels that parallel the arteries mentioned in the previous section (arterial supply). For example, the **temporal veins** (frontal and parietal branches) are found near the temporal arteries and drain into the **retromandibular vein** located posterior to the ramus of the mandible. Also, the **maxillary vein** returns venous blood from the deep face to the retromandibular vein, and the **external and internal jugular veins**. **Facial veins** return blood to the internal jugular vein. Taken together, the facial vein and retromandibular veins drain the face and scalp into the jugular network.

What is the parotid gland? What is its function? What nerves innervate it?

The **parotid glands** are located adjacent to the mandibular rami and secrete saliva into the oral cavity **(see figure 5-1)**. Sensory input (e.g., visual, gustatory, olfactory, appetite) can stimulate the parotid glands via the parasympathetic nervous system to help prepare or facilitate digestion of food within the oral cavity. Parasympathetic fibers of the **glossopharyngeal nerve** (CN IX) increase the secretomotor activity of the parotid gland via the **auriculotemporal nerve** (CN V3; more detail in the Parasympathetics and Ganglion section. Parotid gland secretions drain via the **parotid duct**, which projects anteriorly and pierces the buccinator muscle before entering the oral cavity. A superficial connective tissue layer, called the **parotid sheath**, envelopes the parotid gland and is innervated by the great auricular nerve (C2, C3). Infections of the parotid gland, called **mumps**, produce extreme discomfort while chewing food or speaking. Tumors of the parotid gland occur in approximately 80% of salivary gland cases and are usually benign. During surgical removal of a parotid gland tumor, the facial nerve plexus and subsequent branches are at risk for damage due to their close proximity with the parotid gland.

What are the 5 layers of the SCALP?

The **scalp** covers the calvaria (or cap) of the skull and is described as having five layers. The most superficial **skin** layer typically contains densely packed hair follicles and sebaceous glands. Deep to the skin is a layer of dense **connective tissue** composed of subcutaneous fat, vessels, and nerves. The third layer is an **aponeurosis,** or galea aponeurotica, which spans the frontal and occipital bellies of the occipitofrontalis muscles. A laceration in this layer may produce a gaping wound due to the tension created by these two muscle bellies. This layer assists in preventing the spread of infection because the aponeurosis is continuous with the temporal fascia and attaches to the zygomatic arches, and because the occipital belly attaches to the occipital bone. However, infections can spread anteriorly since the frontalis belly does not attach to the frontal bone, but rather inserts on the orbicularis oculi muscle and skin. A fourth layer of **loose connective tissue** provides a plane of flexibility for the scalp. The scalp can be separated in this layer if a patient experiences accidental scalping, or removal of the scalp from the skull. The deepest layer is the **pericranium,** which resides directly on the surface of the skull bone. In summary, the acronym, SCALP, represents the five layers present from superficial to deep.

What is the trigeminal nerve (CN V)? What are its major branches (CN V1, V2, V3), minor branches? Where are trigeminal nerve and its branches located? What are their functions?

The **trigeminal nerve** (CN V) provides cutaneous sensation over the anterior half of the head. It has three major divisions: the **ophthalmic branch** (V1)**,** the **maxillary branch** (V2)**,** and the **mandibular branch** (V3)**.** Note that each branch is located near regions of the skull associated with its name. The ophthalamic branch exits superficially from the skull near the superior-medial orbital ridge. It divides into the **supraorbital nerve** (a lateral distal branch, via the supraorbital foramen) and **supratrochlear nerve** (a medial distal branch, with no foramen or orbital ridge). Both branches help convey sensory information from the frontal aspect of the skull. Other branches serve cutaneous territory over the nose (e.g., the infratrochlear nerve for the external nasal region). The maxillary branch is distributed to the skin over the middle and anterior face via the **infraorbital nerve,** which exits from the infraorbital foramen. Several branches of the **superior alveolar nerve** of V2 (anterior, middle, and posterior branches) innervates the upper row of teeth. Additional branches serve the zygomatic region (i.e., zygomaticotemporal and zygomaticofacial nerves). The mandibular branch provides cutaneous sensation over the temporal, auricular, buccal (cheek), and mandibular regions. An **auriculotemporal branch** conveys sensory input from the temporal and auricular regions. This branch also carries postsynaptic parasympathetic fibers from the glossopharyngeal nerve (CN IX) destined for the parotid gland. V3 also innervates muscles of mastication including the masseter, temporalis and the pterygoid muscles. Inside the oral cavity, the general sensation of the anterior two thirds of the tongue is conveyed by the **lingual nerve**, a branch of V3. This branch also carries both presynaptic parasympathetic fibers and special taste sensory fibers from the facial nerve (CN VII). The **inferior alveolar nerve** of V3 supplies the mandibular row of teeth are supplied, and terminates distally over the mental protuberance (i.e., chin) as the mental nerve, via the mental foramen. A **buccal branch** of V3 innervates the lateral wall of the oral cavity (cheek).

See CM 5-2A, 5-2B, 5-2C, 5-2D, 5-2E, and 5-2F for Review.

CM 5-2A

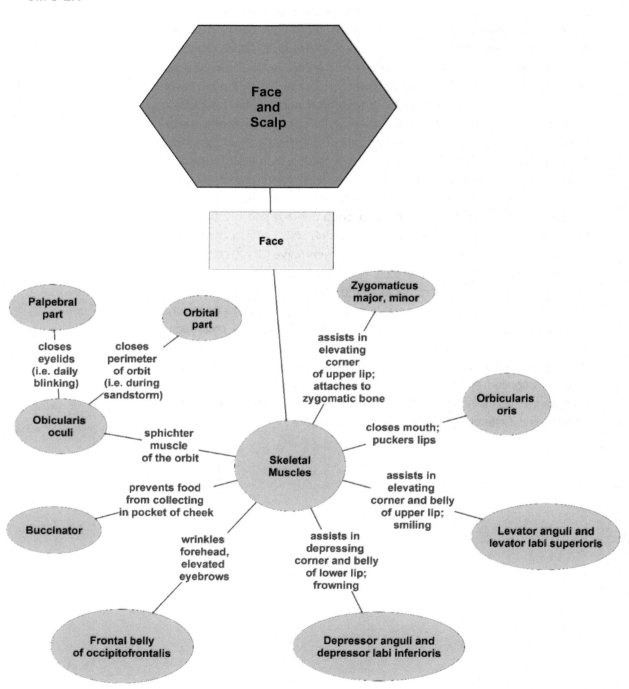

CM 5-2B

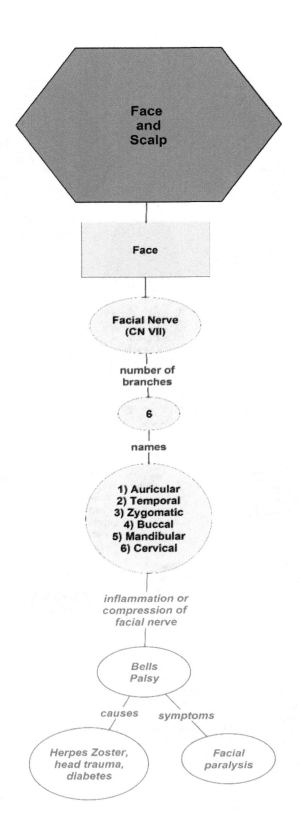

CM 5-2C

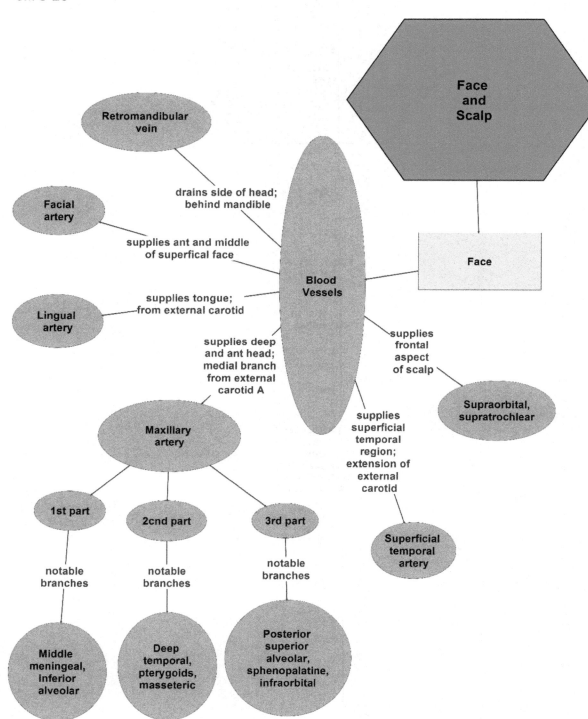

Face and Scalp

Blood Vessels

Face

Retromandibular vein — drains side of head; behind mandible

Facial artery — supplies ant and middle of superfical face

Lingual artery — supplies tongue; from external carotid

supplies deep and ant head; medial branch from external carotid A — Maxillary artery

supplies frontal aspect of scalp — Supraorbital, supratrochlear

supplies superficial temporal region; extension of external carotid — Superficial temporal artery

Maxillary artery → 1st part → notable branches → Middle meningeal, Inferior alveolar

Maxillary artery → 2cnd part → notable branches → Deep temporal, pterygoids, masseteric

Maxillary artery → 3rd part → notable branches → Posterior superior alveolar, sphenopalatine, infraorbital

CM 5-2D

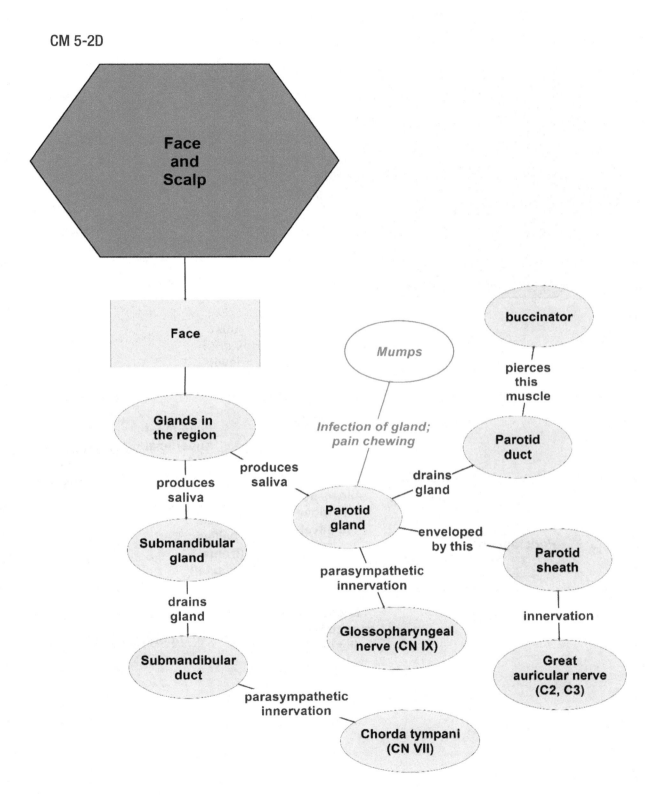

CM 5-2E

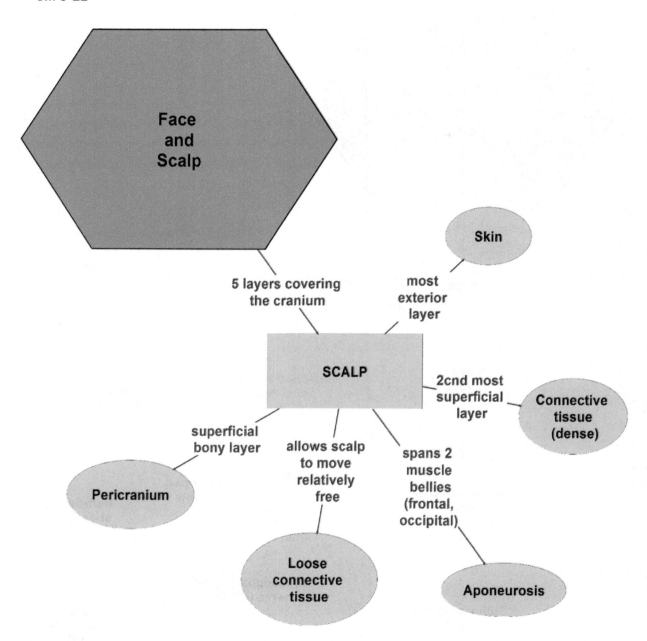

CM 5-2F

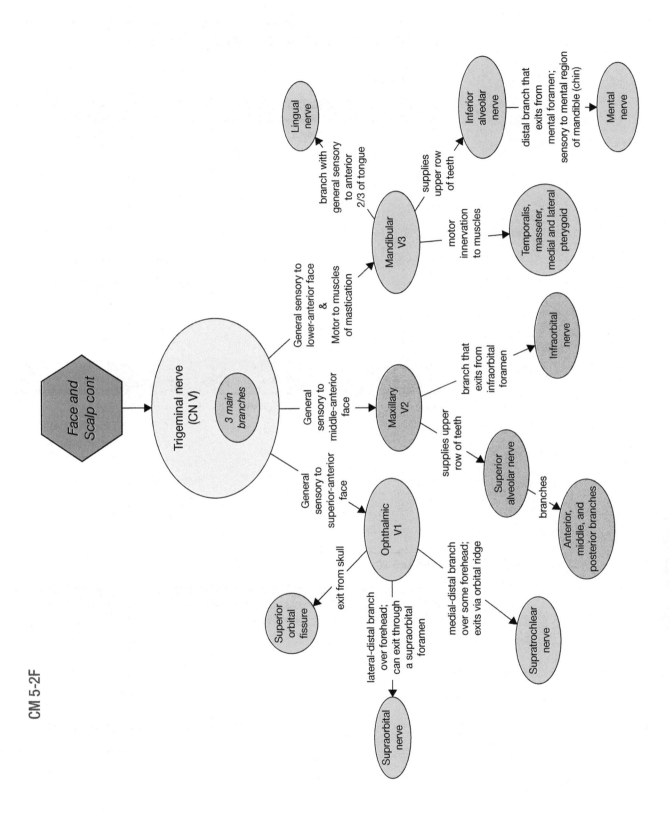

Synthesis Exercise: Create a concept map using items from EXERCISE 5-2A, 5-2B, 5-2C, 5-2D, 5-2E, and 5-2F.

Exercise 5-2A

Primary Category	Secondary Categories	Continuations
Face	Skeletal muscles	Frontal belly of occipitofrontalis
		Buccinator
		Orbicularis oculi
		Orbital part
		Palpebral part
		Zygomaticus major, minor
		Orbicularis oris
		Levator anguli, levator labi superioris
		Depressor anguli and depressor labi inferioris

Exercise 5-2B

Primary Category	Secondary Categories	Continuations	Clinical Considerations
Face	Facial nerve (CN VII)	6	Bells Palsy
		Auricular	Facial Paralysis
		Temporal	Herpes zoster virus, head trauma, diabetes
		Zygomatic	
		Buccal	
		Mandibular	
		Cervical	

Exercise 5-2C

Primary Category	Secondary Categories	Continuations
Face	Blood vessels	Superficial temporal artery
		Supraorbital, supratrochlear
		Maxillary artery
		1st part
		2nd part
		3rd part
		Posterior superior alveolar
		Sphenopalantine

Primary Category	Secondary Categories	Continuations
		Infraorbital
		Deep temporal
		Pterygoids
		Masseteric
		Middle meningeal
		Inferior alveolar
		Lingual
		Facial
		Retromandibular vein

Exercise 5-2D

Primary Category	Secondary Categories	Continuations	Clinical Considerations
Face	Glands in the region	Parotid gland	Mumps
		Parotid duct	
		Buccinator	
		Parotid sheath	
		Greater auricular nerve (C2, C3)	
		Glossopharyngeal nerve (CN IX)	
		Submandibular duct	
		Chorda tympani (CN VII)	

Exercise 5-2E

Primary Category	Secondary Categories
SCALP	Skin
	Connective tissue (dense)
	Aponeurosis
	Loose connective tissue
	Pericranium

Exercise 5-2F

Primary Category	Secondary Categories	Continuations
Trigeminal nerve (CN V)	Ophthalmic V1	Superior orbital fissure
	Maxillary V2	Supraorbital nerve
	Mandibular V3	Supratrochlear nerve
		Superior alveolar nerve
		Infraorbital nerve
		Anterior, middle, posterior branches
		Lingual nerve
		Inferior alveolar nerve
		Mental nerve
		Temporalis
		Masseter
		Medial and lateral pterygoid

III. Cranial Cavity and Brain

Overview of key topics for this section:

- Cranial meninges
- Middle meningeal artery
- Dural folds
- Venous sinuses and drainage
- Production of cerebrospinal fluid
- Gross anatomy of the brain
- Epidural, subdural, and subarachnoid hematomas

What are the three layers of cranial meninges?

Three protective membranes surround the brain. These are primarily continuous with the spinal cord meninges and thus collectively envelop the central nervous system. The **dura mater** (from the Latin for *tough mother)* is the most external layer of meninges and can be divided into two additional layers: the **external periosteal layer**, which lines the periosteum of the skull, and the **internal meningeal layer**, which is continuous with the dura of the spinal cord. The superior sagittal sinus is located between these two layers of dura mater. The middle layer of meninges, the **arachnoid mater** (from the Latin for *spider-like*), creates web-like projections in the subarachnoid space. **Cerebrospinal fluid** fills the **subarachnoid space** and bathes the central nervous system. Several pockets of arachnoid, called **arachnoid granulations,** traverse the dura mater into the superior sagittal sinus. At this specific location, cerebrospinal fluid can be recycled into the venous system. The arachnoid granulations create small pits on the internal aspect of the skull, called **granular fovea**. The deepest layer of meninges, closest to the brain, is the **pia mater** (from the Latin for *tender mother")*. This layer envelopes many blood vessels on the surface of the brain. **Leptomeninges** refers to both the arachnoid and pia mater. Bacterial or viral infections of the meninges can cause inflammation leading to **meningitis**.

What is the middle meningeal artery?

The primary arterial supply to the dura mater is the **middle meningeal artery**. It arises from the first part of the maxillary artery, ascends into the skull via the foramen spinosum, and divides into anterior and posterior branches. The anterior branch usually courses deep to the pterion of the skull and can be damaged by trauma (more detail in a later section).

What are the four primary dural folds?

Dura mater invaginates the brain in four specific areas as **dural folds**. The **falx cerebri (**or **cerebral falx)** is located between the right and left cerebral hemispheres **(see figure 5-5)**. It spans from the **crita galli** to the internal occipital protuberance of the skull **(see figure 5-5)**. Within the falx cerebri is the **inferior sagittal sinus** for venous drainage. The **falx cerebelli (**or **cerebellar falx)** separates the right and left cerebellum. Superior to the cerebellum and inferior to the occipital lobe of the cerebrum is the **tentorium cerebelli (**or **cerebellar tentorium) (see figure 5-5)**. Another dural fold, called the **diaphragm sellae (**or **sellar diaphragm),** lies just superior to the **sella turcica**. It serves as the immediate roof of the pituitary gland. However, a single circular hole in this dural fold allows passage of the

Figure 5-5

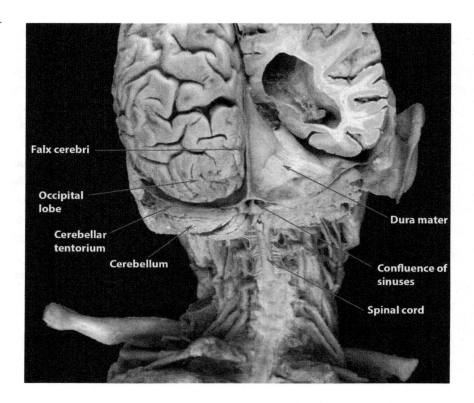

Falx cerebri

Occipital lobe

Cerebellar tentorium

Cerebellum

Dura mater

Confluence of sinuses

Spinal cord

pituitary stalk (or infundibulum). Meningeal branches of the trigeminal nerve (CN V) innverate a significant portion of the dural folds.

What are the venous sinuses in the skull? What is path of venous drainage?

Several **venous sinuses**, or blood vessels containing venous blood, are distributed within the cranial cavity. Located in the midline of the skull, three venous sinuses drain blood from anterior to posterior: (1) the **superior sagittal sinus, which is the** largest and the most superior; (2) the **inferior sagittal sinus,** which lies just inferior; and (3) the **great cerebral vein,** which is small and more inferior. The inferior sagittal sinus and the great cerebral vein both drain into a short canal called the **straight sinus**. Anterior to the internal occipital protuberance, the **confluence of sinuses** receives venous blood from the straight sinus and the superior sagittal sinus (**see figure 5-5**). At this location, blood is distributed bilaterally to the **transverse sinuses** (within the transverse groove) and subsequently to the **sigmoid sinus** (within the sigmoid groove). The terminal aspect of the sigmoid sinus exits the skull via the **jugular foramen** and becomes the **internal jugular vein**. Additionally, venous blood from the face can be drain into the cranial cavity through the superior and inferior **ophthalmic veins**. This pathway drains into the **cavernous sinus** which is a venous reservoir surrounding the **sella turcica** of the skull. The pituitary gland, internal carotid arteries, and several cranial nerves are located adjacent to or within the cavernous sinus. Blood exits the cavernous sinus through two pathways: through the sigmoid sinus via the **superior petrosal sinus,** or through the jugular foramen by way of the **inferior petrosal sinus**.

Where is cerebrospinal fluid produced? What is its function?

The choroid plexus of the four ventricles (two lateral ventricles, the third, and the fourth ventricle) in the brain helps produce cerebrospinal fluid (CSF). The CNS houses approximately 125 milliliters of CSF, which is replenished about four times per day. Thus, the choroid plexus produces about 0.5 L per day. CSF in the subarachnoid space is recycled into the superior sagittal sinus via arachnoid granulations. The function of CSF is to buffer or cushion movement of the brain inside the cranial cavity. Also, it may help flush out metabolic toxins or waste products from the brain. Significant reductions in CSF volume due to diuretic consumption (alcohol) may produce headaches.

What are the surface features and gross anatomy of the brain? What are some unique functions of each region?

The **cerebrum** is separated into four major lobes with **gyri** (ridges) and **sulci** (depressions). It is also divided into bilateral cerebral hemispheres (right and left) via the **longitudinal fissure**. The **frontal lobes** are found anterior in the cranial cavity. The central sulcus separates frontal lobes from **parietal lobes,** which is a superior-posterior aspect of the cerebrum. Immediately anterior to the central sulcus is the **primary motor cortex** of the frontal lobe. Immediately posterior to the central sulcus is the **primary somatosensory cortex** of the parietal lobe. The **temporal lobes** of the cerebrum resides laterally in the cranial cavity and promote visual memories as well as language. The **occipital lobes** of the cerebrum are located posteriorly and inferiorly in the cranial cavity **(see figure 5-5)**, and serve as a visual processing center. The **cerebellum** resides inferior to the occipital lobe of the cerebrum **(see figure 5-5)**. The most established function of the cerebellum is proprioception and coordination of motor movements. The **diencephalon** of the forebrain, comprised of the thalamus, hypothalamus, and epithalamus, is located deep and central in the brain. Functionally, the diencephalon helps control substantial endocrine function. The brain stem has three major parts. The **mid-brain or mesencephalon,** just inferior to the diencephalon, is associated with the oculomotor nerve (CN III) and the trochlear nerve (CN IV). The **pons,** located between the mid-brain (superior) and the medulla oblongata (inferior), is associated with the trigeminal nerve (CN V). Lastly, the medulla oblongata is most inferior part of the brain stem and is associated with the glossopharyngeal nerve (CN IX), vagus nerve (CN X), and hypoglossal nerve (CN XII). The facial nerve (CN VII) and vestibulo-cochlear nerve (CN VIII) are associated with the junction of the pons and the medulla oblongata.

What is an epidural hematoma? What is a dural border hematoma? What is a subarachnoid hematoma?

Injuries to blood vessels wall within the cranial cavity can lead to hematomas, or blood pooling. An **epidural hematoma** often occurs following damage to the middle meningeal artery. Blood collects superficial to the dura mater and deep to the skull. Common causes include blunt trauma to the lateral aspect of the skull at the pterion (e.g., baseball impact). A **dural border** or **subdural hematoma** occurs between the dura mater and the arachnoid mater. In this event, a potential space becomes a real space. Causes include damaged cerebral veins due to high acceleration or deceleration of the head (e.g., car accident). A subarachnoid hematoma occurs during damage to a cerebral artery whereby blood collects in the subarachnoid space. An aneurysm, or localized weakening of an arterial wall is common among subarachnoid hematomas.

See CM 5-3A, 5-3B, and 5-3C for Review.

CM 5-3A

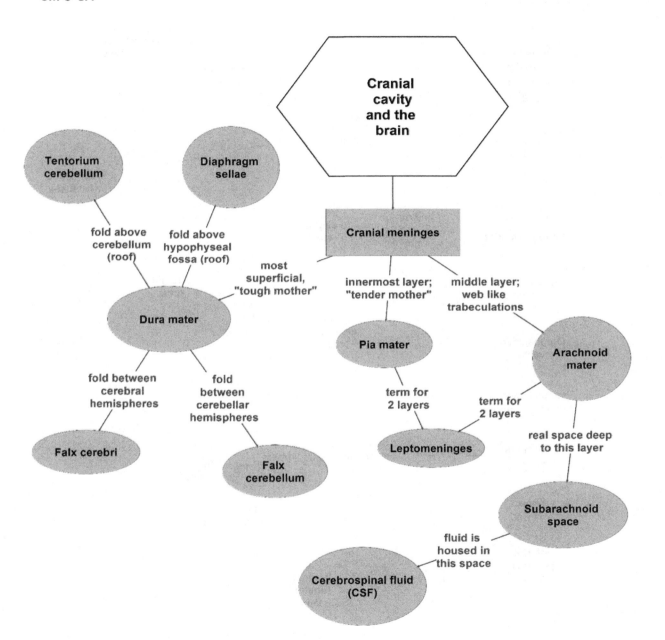

CM 5-3B

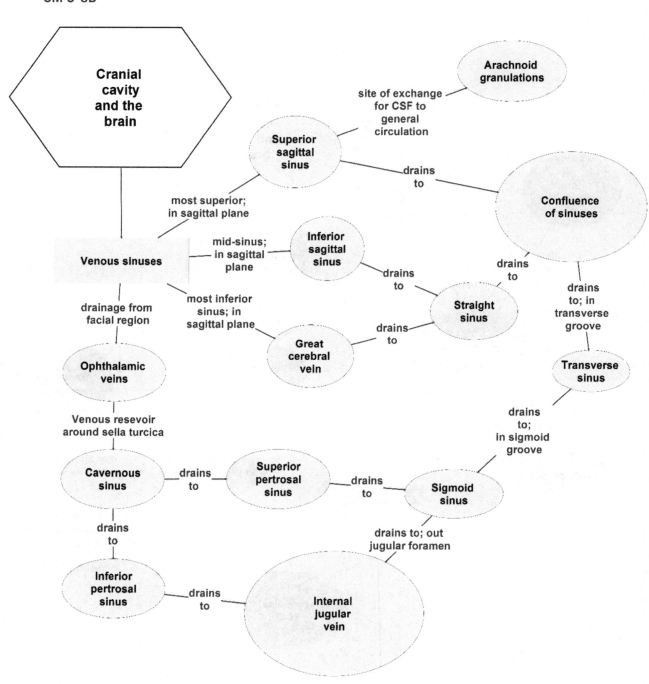

Cranial cavity and the brain

Arachnoid granulations

site of exchange for CSF to general circulation

Superior sagittal sinus

drains to

Confluence of sinuses

most superior; in sagittal plane

Venous sinuses

mid-sinus; in sagittal plane

Inferior sagittal sinus

drains to

drains to

drains to; in transverse groove

most inferior sinus; in sagittal plane

Straight sinus

drains to

Transverse sinus

drainage from facial region

Great cerebral vein

drains to

Ophthalamic veins

Venous resevoir around sella turcica

drains to; in sigmoid groove

Cavernous sinus

drains to

Superior pertrosal sinus

drains to

Sigmoid sinus

drains to

drains to; out jugular foramen

Inferior pertrosal sinus

drains to

Internal jugular vein

CM 5-3C

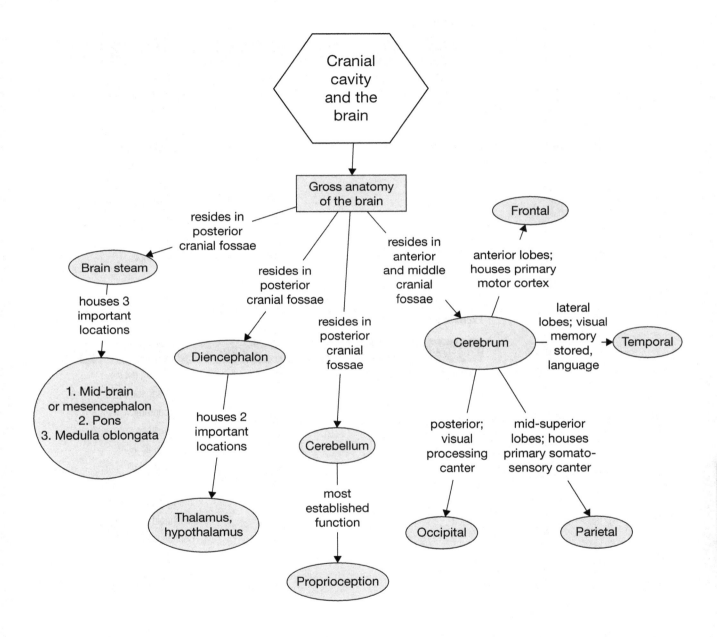

Synthesis Exercise: Create a concept map using items from EXERCISE 5-3A, 5-3B, and 5-3C.

Exercise 5-3A

Primary Category	Secondary Category	Continuations
Cranial cavity and the brain	Cranial meninges	Dura mater
		Falx cerebellum
		Falx cerebri
		Tentorium cerebellum
		Diaphragm sellae
		Arachnoid mater
		Subarachnoid space
		Cerebrospinal fluid (CSF)
		Choroid plexus
		Pia mater
		Leptomeninges

Exercise 5-3B

Primary Category	Secondary Category	Continuations
Cranial cavity and the brain	Venous sinuses	Superior sagittal sinus
		Inferior sagittal sinus
		Great cerebral vein
		Straight sinus
		Ophthalamic veins
		Cavernous sinus
		Superior petrosal vein
		Inferior petrosal vein
		Arachnoid granulations
		Confluence of sinuses
		Transverse sinus
		Sigmoid sinus
		Internal jugular vein

Exercise 5-3C

Primary Category	Secondary Category	Continuations
Cranial cavity and the brain	Gross anatomy of the brain	Brain stem
		Diencephalon
		Cerebellum
		Cerebrum
		Mid-brain or mesencephalon
		Pons
		Medulla oblongata
		Thalamus
		Hypothalamus
		Proprioception
		Frontal
		Parietal
		Temporal
		Occipital

IV. The Eye

Overview of key topics for this section:

- The orbit
- Surface anatomy of the eye
- Lacrimal fluid production and drainage
- Anatomy of the eyeball
- Shape change of iris and lens
- Extraocular muscles and movements
- Occulomotor and abducens nerve paralysis

What bones produce the orbit? What are its unique features?

The orbit houses the eye and is composed of several bones. The anterior bones include the frontal (superior), maxillary (inferior), and zygomatic (lateral).

The posterior bones include the lacrimal (medial), ethmoid (central), and sphenoid (lateral). The **optic canal** (for the optic nerve), **superior orbital fissure** (for CN III, IV, V1 , VI), and **inferior orbital fissure** (for CV V2) are located posteriorly in the sphenoid bone of the orbit. Other unique bony features include the **lacrimal groove** for the lacrimal sac of the lacrimal bone and the **supraorbital notch,** or foramen for the supraorbital artery and nerve.

What are the surface anatomy features of the orbit and eye?

The superior and inferior **eyelids (or palpebra)** are thin layers of skin covering the eye. They provide a protective function for the underlying eyeball and also help pass lacrimal fluid over the superficial surface of the eyeball from lateral to medial (i.e. blinking). **Bulbar conjunctiva** and **palpebral conjunctiva**, layers of stratified squamous epithelia, covers the internal aspect of the eyelids and the surface of the sclera, respectively. The **lacrimal punctum** for fluid drainage are openings on the medial aspect of the upper and lower eyelids. **Sclera** is an external layer of fibrous tissue that covers the eyeball and contributes to the white aspect of the eye. The **iris** and **pupil** are in the center of the eye. The iris can be different colors in different individuals due to differing pigmentation. Muscles that act on the iris control the size of its hollow opening, or pupil. The function of the pupil is to control how much light enters the eyeball. For example, dilation of the pupil occurs in dim or dark settings while the pupil becomes constricted in bright settings (more details later).

Where is lacrimal fluid produced and drained?

Lacrimal fluid is produced by the lacrimal gland, located in the deep superior-lateral aspect of the orbit. Once produced, the lacrimal fluid flows across the surface of the eyeball into the **lacrimal punctum, lacrimal canaliculi, lacrimal sac,** and **nasolacrimal duct**. Functionally, this drainage system terminates in the nasal cavity.

What is the eyeball and its underlying anatomy?

The eyeball is a spherical structure for vision that resides in the orbit of skull. Orbital fat buffers the eyeball from external forces or acceleration of the head. The most anterior layer of the eyeball is the **cornea,** which begins the refraction of light for the retina and subsequent visual processing. It receives nutrients via diffusion from both lacrimal fluid and aqueous humor. The **anterior chamber** is immediately posterior to the cornea and anterior to the iris. It houses the aqueous humor, which helps maintain intraocular pressure. The **iris and pupil** change shape to control the amount of light hitting the **retina**. The **lens** resides posterior to the iris and helps further refract or focus light onto the retina. Tension from the attached **zonular fibers** can change the shape of the lens via contraction or relaxation. The lens flattens for distant object focusing and becomes spherical for near object focusing. The **ciliary body**, near and around the circumference of the lens. It contains muscles that help create tension for the zonular fibers of the lens. In addition, the ciliary body is the site of aqueous humor production, which distributes to the anterior chamber. The **posterior segment** is a large cavity of the eyeball located posterior to the lens. It contains a jelly-like substance called **vitreous humor**, which helps prevent the eyeball from collapsing and serves as a translucent medium for light to pass through to the retina. The eyeball has three layers: (1) the **retina** (deep), (2) the **choroid** (middle), and (3) the **sclera** (superficial). Special photoreceptor cells (**rods** and **cones**) in the retina enable visual perception. The optic nerve (CN II), which leaves the retina at a site that lacks photoreceptors called the optic disc, transmits electrical impulses from the retina to the brain. The highly vascularized choroid layer of the eyeball is continuous with the ciliary body and iris anteriorly. Arterial supply to the eye is via the **ophthalmic artery**, **posterior ciliary arteries** (approximately eight), and the **posterior retinal artery**. The sclera layer of the eyeball is fibrous and provides a strong protective wall for the eyeball. It is continuous with the cornea anteriorly.

What is glaucoma? What is a cataract?

Glaucoma is an eye disease that results in a size reduction of the visual field. It occurs slowly over time and thought to develop via increased pressure inside the eyeball (intraocular pressure). The mechanism is described as either **open angle** or **closed angle glaucoma**. Open angle glaucoma results from slow exit of aqueous humor through the **trabecular mesh**. Although the etiology of open angle glaucoma is not established, the iris does *not* physically obstruct the exit of aqueous humor. In closed angle glaucoma, the iris blocks the trabecular mesh and the outflow of aqueous humor. In both types, the poor drainage of aqueous humor leads to elevated intraocular pressure, compression of the retina, and a reduction in the visual field. If left untreated, blindness may ensue. A **cataract** is the blurring of vision due to a less transparent lens, which can be described as cloudiness. Aging and the breakdown of the lens tissue can contribute to cataracts. Surgery can be used for correction of this type of eye disease.

What is the pupillary reflex of the eye? What is the accommodation reflex?

Autonomic reflexes of the eye allow changes in pupil size (**pupillary reflex**) and the shape of the lens (**accommodation**). The pupillary reflex is controlled by both parasympathetic and sympathetic innervation. During bright light, parasympathetic nerves stimulate the **sphincter pupillae muscles** to decreases the size of the pupil, allowing less light to enter the eyeball. In dim lighting (e.g., dark room), sympathetic nerves stimulate the **dilator pupillae** muscles to increase the size of the pupil, allowing more light to enter the eyeball. Similar dilation of the pupil occurs during a **fight or flight response** due to increased sympathetic nervous system activity. Accommodation is a reflex that controls the shape of the lens and serves to improve focus by optimally refracting (or focusing) light onto the retina. For example, the lens changes shape for focus of images at a long distance versus a short distance. However, it relies only on parasympathetic innervation of the ciliary muscles. Sympathetic innervation does not occur in this reflex. The lens prefers a spherical shape and moves toward this shape. During focus of near objects, parasympathetic nerve activity changes the shape of the lens to become more spherical. As a result, the ciliary muscles contract and the zonular fibers relax. In contrast, when focusing on distant objects, the shape of the lens flattens due to decreased parasympathetic stimulation. Consequently, the ciliary muscles relax and the zonular fibers contract. Without tension from the attached zonular fibers, the lens shape becomes flatter.

What is myopia? What is presbyopia?

Myopia (i.e., near-sightedness) produces blurred vision of distant objects, but near vision is clear. The mechanism includes an eyeball that is too long. Thus, light from distant objects is refracted in front of the retina, appearing blurry. In contrast, **presbyopia** (i.e., far-sightedness) produces blurred vision of near objects, but normal vision of distant objects. Aging is a key risk factor for presbyopia. The mechanism involves the gradual hardening and flattening of the lens. The flatter lens fails to refract light of near objects directly onto the lens and instead, refracts the light beyond the retina.

What is gaze? What are the three axes of movement? How is the gaze of the eyeball shifted by specific extraocular muscles from a primary position? What is its innervation?

Gaze is a specific directional aim of the pupil. In the primary position (anatomical position), it is centrally placed and pointed anteriorly. Movements of the eye occur in three axes, which are (1) the vertical axis for abduction-adduction, (2) the transverse axis for elevation and depression, and (3) the anterior-posterior axis for lateral and medial rotation. **Extraocular muscles** can act on the eyeball to alter gaze for tracking objects within the visual field. Muscles can work together to facilitate a specific movement. For example, the primary movers create the most significant action and secondary movers assist the primary movers. Also, two eye muscles, called **synergists**, perform a specific movement starting from the primary position. Thus, synergistic movements differ from clinical testing of a single muscle. Note: all of the movements describe below occur starting from the primary position and do not reflect the clinical testing of a specific muscle. Elevation of the eyelid is produced by contraction of the **levator palpebrae superioris muscle**. It is an extraocular muscle that does not influence the gaze. A **common tendinous ring** is located in the posterior aspect of the orbit and serves as a common attachment site for several of the extraocular muscles.

Adduction versus Abduction: The primary mover for adduction is the **medial rectus muscle** with secondary movement by the **superior rectus** and **inferior rectus muscles**. The **lateral rectus muscle** is the primary mover for abduction with secondary movement by the **superior** and inferior **oblique muscles**.

Elevation versus Depression: Elevation of gaze requires synergistic action of the superior rectus and inferior oblique muscles. Depression of gaze requires synergistic action of the inferior rectus and superior oblique muscles.

Medial versus Lateral Rotators: **Intorsion** (medial rotation towards the nose using high noon) occurs via either superior rectus or superior oblique muscles. **Extorsion** (lateral rotation away from the nose using high noon) relies on either the inferior rectus or inferior oblique muscle. Movements of intorsion and extortion are relatively minor.

Finally, cranial nerves III, IV, VI innervate the extraocular muscles (see below).

- Lateral rectus: abducens nerve, CN VI
- Superior oblique: trochlear nerve, CN IV
- Levator palbebrae superioris: oculomotor nerve, CN III
- Superior rectus: oculomotor nerve, CN III
- Medial rectus: oculomotor nerve, CN III
- Inferior rectus: oculomotor nerve, CN III
- Inferior oblique: oculomotor nerve, CN III

$LR_6SO_4AO_3$ is a convenient learning mnemonic for eye muscles and innervations: (**L**ateral **R**ectus **6** (VI), **S**uperior **O**blique **4** (IV), **A**ll **O**thers **3** (III).

What deficits occur following oculomotor (CN III) palsy?
What deficits occur following abducens nerve (CN VI) palsy?

Paralysis of the extraocular muscles can occur due to nerve palsy. Risk factors include head trauma or injury. For example, oculomotor nerve (CN III) palsy results in a gaze pointed inferiorly and laterally due to unopposed action of the lateral rectus (CN VI) and superior oblique (CN IV) muscles. In addition, a droopy eyelid may be present due to lack of the levator palpebrae superioris muscle. Abducens nerve (CN VI) palsy results in gaze pointing medially due to unopposed action of medial rectus muscle (CN III). Double vision (or diplopia) usually occurs when a patient with palsy of CN III or CN IV attempts to use the associated eye muscles.

See CM 5-4A, 5-4B, 5-4C, 5-4D, and 5-4E for Review.

CM 5-4A

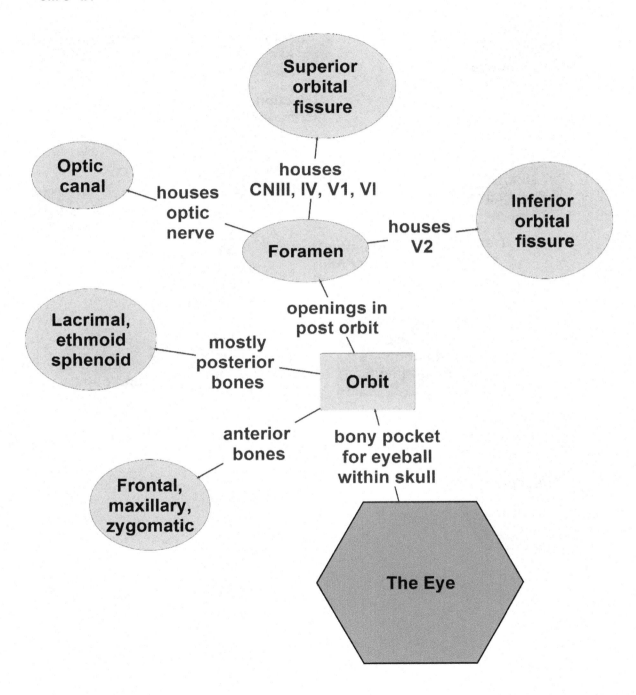

CM 5-4B

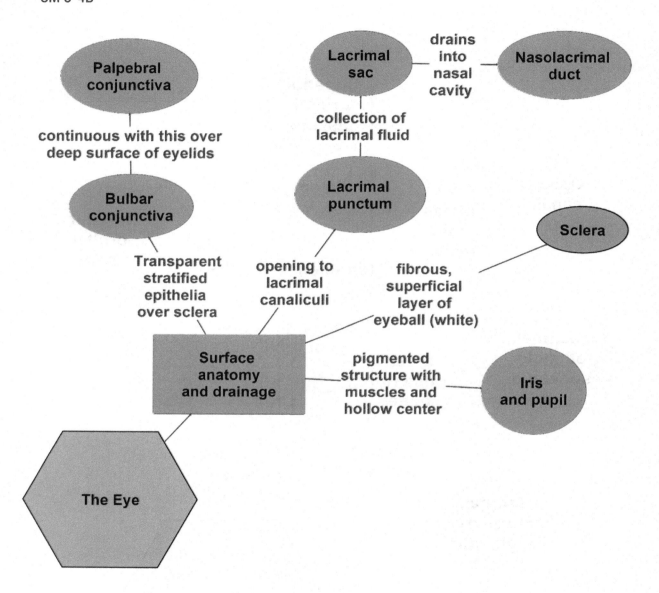

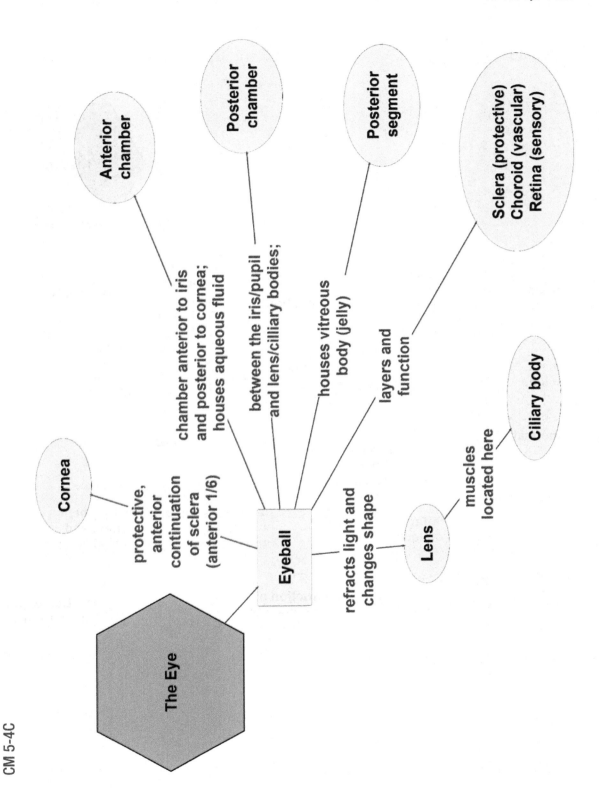

CM 5-4C

The Eye

Eyeball

Cornea
— protective, anterior continuation of sclera (anterior 1/6)

Anterior chamber
— chamber anterior to iris and posterior to cornea; houses aqueous fluid

Posterior chamber
— between the iris/pupil and lens/cilliary bodies;

Posterior segment
— houses vitreous body (jelly)

**Sclera (protective)
Choroid (vascular)
Retina (sensory)**
— layers and function

Lens
— refracts light and changes shape

Ciliary body
— muscles located here

CM 5-4D

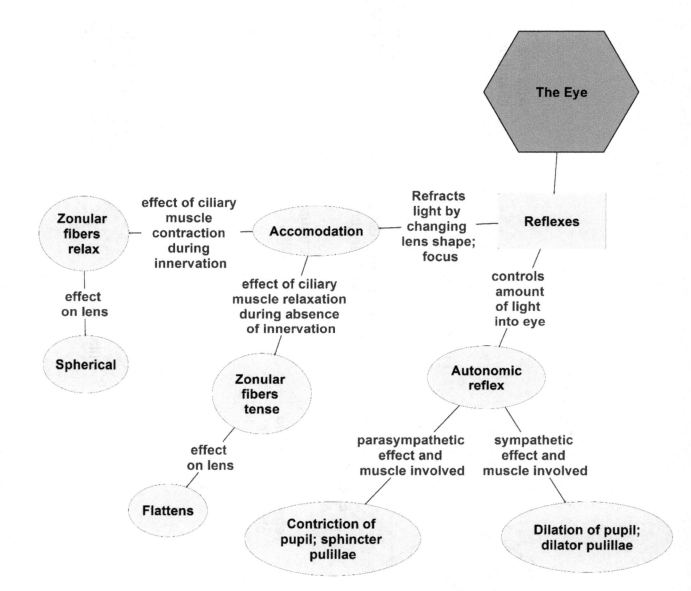

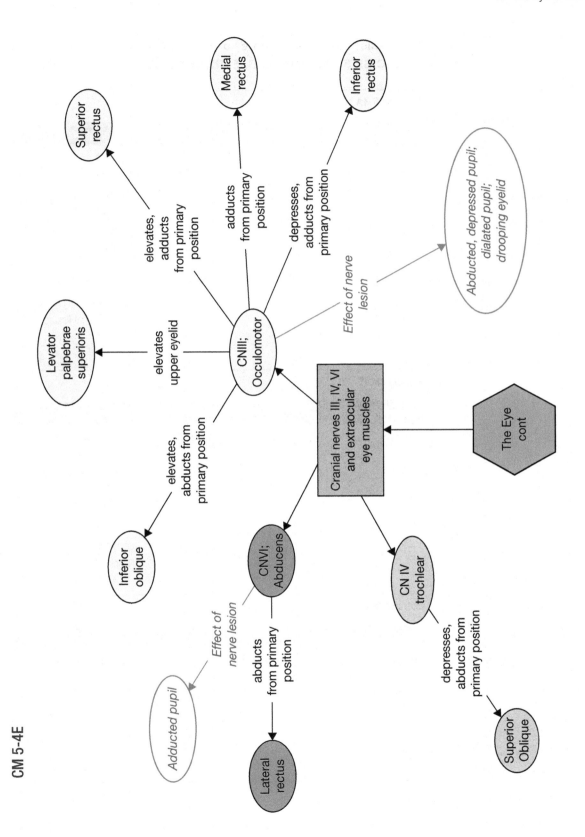

CM 5-4E

Synthesis Exercise: Create a concept map using items from EXERCISE 5-4A, 5-4B, 5-4C, 5-4D, and 5-4E.

Exercise 5-4A

Primary Category	Secondary Category	Continuations
The Eye	Orbit	Foramen
		Lacrimal
		Ethmoid
		Sphenoid
		Frontal
		Maxillary
		Zygomatic
		Optic canal
		Superior orbital fissure
		Inferior orbital fissure

Exercise 5-4B

Primary Category	Secondary Category	Continuations
The Eye	Surface anatomy and drainage	Bulbar conjunctiva
		Lacrimal punctum
		Sclera
		Iris
		Pupil
		Palpebral conjunctiva
		Lacrimal sac
		Nasolacrimal duct

Exercise 5-4C

Primary Category	Secondary Category	Continuations
The Eye	The eyeball	Sclera
		Iris
		Pupil
		Lens
		Cornea
		Cillary body
		Anterior chamber

Primary Category	Secondary Category	Continuations
		Posterior chamber
		Posterior segment
		Sclera (protective)
		Choroid (vascular)
		Retina (sensory)

Exercise 5-4D

Primary Category	Secondary Categories	Continuations
The Eye	Reflexes	Accommodation
		Autonomic reflex
		Zonular fibers relax
		Zonular fibers tense
		Spherical
		Flattens
		Contraction of pupil; sphincter pupillae
		Dilation of pupil; dilator pupillae

Exercise 5-4E

Primary Category	Secondary Categories	Continuations	Clinical Considerations
The Eye	Cranial nerves III, IV, VI and extraocular eye muscles	CN III; oculomotor	Abducted, depressed pupil
		CN IV; trochlear	Dilated pupil
		CN VI; abducens	Drooping eyelid
		Inferior oblique	Adducted pupil
		Levator palpebrae superioris	
		Superior rectus	
		Medial rectus	
		Inferior rectus	
		Superior oblique	
		Lateral rectus	

V. Skull — Part II

Overview of key topics for this section:

- Paranasal sinuses
- Anterior, middle, and posterior cranial fossas
- Sites of entry and exit of cranial nerve or vessels from the skull

What are the four paranasal sinuses? What is a sinus infection?

The skull contains four pairs of small, air-filled pockets adjacent to the nasal cavity called paranasal sinuses. These include the maxillary sinuses (embedded in the maxillary bone inferior to the orbit), the frontal sinuses (within the frontal bone superior to the orbit), the ethmoidal sinsuses (within the ethmoid bone, or ethmoidal air cells), and the sphenoidal sinuses (within the sphenoid bone). In response to a bacterial or allergen, the paranasal sinuses can be blocked and filled with mucus resulting in a sinus infection, or sinusitis. Patients experience a congested feeling in the facial region due to the fluid-filled sinuses and, which promote an accompanying headache.

What are the three cranial fossas of the skull? What are the foramena and accompanying cranial nerves or vessels? What is the path of the internal carotid artery to reach the brain? What unique features are found on the external base of the skull?

The internal base of the cranial cavity can be divided into three hollow areas- the **anterior, middle, and posterior cranial fossas**. The anterior cranial fossa is comprised of the orbital plate of the frontal bone, the cristal galli, cribiform plate and ethmoidal foramina for CN I (the olfactory nerve), and the lesser wing and anterior clinoid processes of the sphenoid bone. Just posterior to the lesser wing of the sphenoid bone sits the middle cranial fossa, divided into a median part and a lateral parts. The sella turcica (or Turkish saddle) is a U-shaped groove within the median part that houses the pituitary gland. The **optic chiasm** is located in the prechiasmatic groove, just anterior to the sella turcica. . Similar to a saddle, the sella turcica has three parts: the tuberculum sellae (the horn of saddle), the hypophysial fossa (the seat of saddle), and the dorsum sellae (the back of saddle). Two optic canals for CN II (optic nerve) sit in the anterior aspect of the middle cranial fossa. The **internal carotid artery** is located immediately lateral to the median part of the sella turcica. The pathway of this major arterial supply to the brain begins with the external opening of the carotid canal, which leads to the carotid canal and the internal opening of the canal. The carotid grooves and anterior clinoid processes are bony features of the skull that help create the arterial pathway for the internal carotid artery which ultimately leads to the cerebral arterial circle, or Circle of Willis **(see figure 5-6)**. Here, the basilar artery and two internal carotid

Figure 5-6

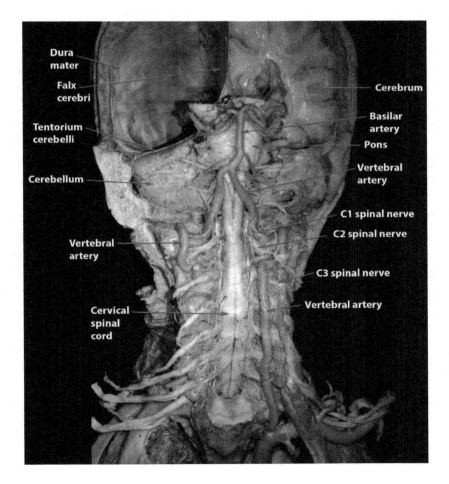

arteries anastomose to supply the anterior, middle, and posterior cerebral arteries. The lateral part of the middle cranial fossa, which primarily houses the temporal lobe of the cerebrum, has the following foramena within the greater wing of the sphenoid bone: (1) the **superior orbital fissure** for the oculomotor, trochlear, and ophthalamic branch of the trigeminal nerve, and the abducens (CN III, IV, V1, and VI, respectively); (2) the **foramen rotundum** for the maxillary nerve of trigeminal (V2); (3) the **foramen ovale** for the mandibular nerve of trigeminal (V3), and (4) the **foramen spinosum** for middle meningeal artery first part of maxillary artery). The remaining lateral part of the middle cranial fossa is composed of temporal bone divided into a squamous part (flat and horizontal) and a petrous part (ridge). The petrous ridge of the temporal bone houses the auditory and vestibular systems (CN VIII, or the vestibulocochlear nerve) of the skull. The posterior cranial fossa is composed primarily of occipital bone, which contains the cerebellum, pons, and medulla oblongata. The tentorium cerebelli dura fold (or cerebellar tentorium), creates the roof of this fossa and separates it from the occipital lobe of the cerebrum. Several foramina are found in the posterior cranial fossa: (1) the **foramen magnum** for the spinal cord, entry of the spinal accessory nerve (CN XI), and vertebral arteries; (2) the **hypoglossal canal** for the hypoglossal nerve (CN XII), (3) the **jugular foramen** for the glossopharyngeal, vagus, and spinal accessory nerves (CN IX, X, and XI), and the beginning of the internal jugular vein), and (4) the **internal acoustic meatus** for the facial and vestibulocochlear nerves (CN VII, VIII). On the external base of the skull, the head of the mandible articulates with the temporal fossa. This joint is just anterior to the stylomastoid foramen, which is an opening for the facial nerve and the styloid process, where muscles and ligaments. A larger tubercle, called the mastoid process, lies just posterior to the external acoustic meatus, which is an attachment site for the sternocleidomastoid muscle. The **basiocciput** with the **pharyngeal tubercles** is found immediately anterior to the foramen magnum, serving as an attachment site for the superior **pharyngeal constrictor muscle**.

See CM 5-5A, 5-5B, 5-5C, and 5-5D for Review.

CM 5-5A

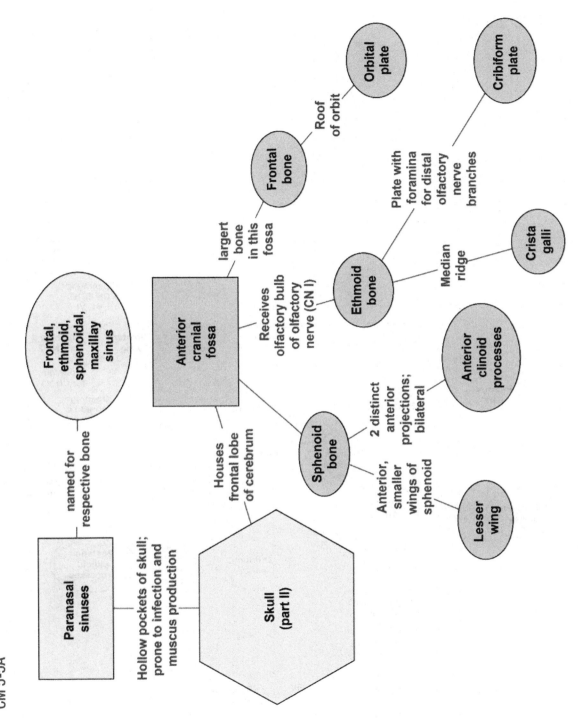

CM 5-5B

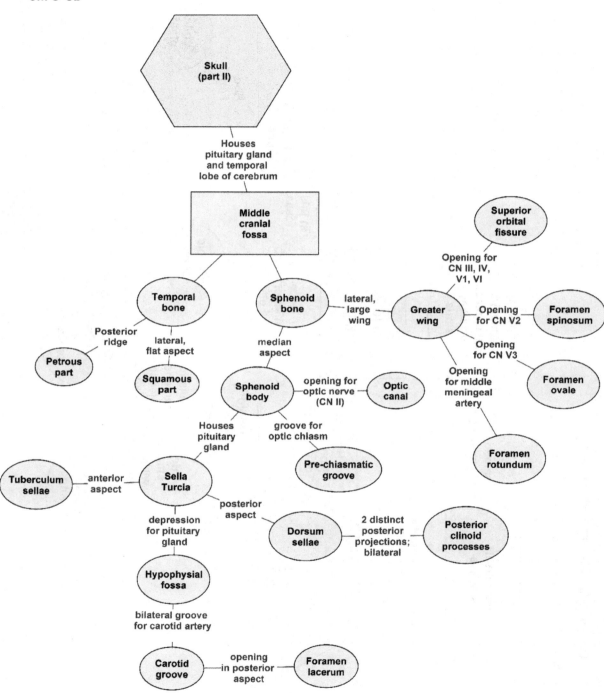

CM 5-5C

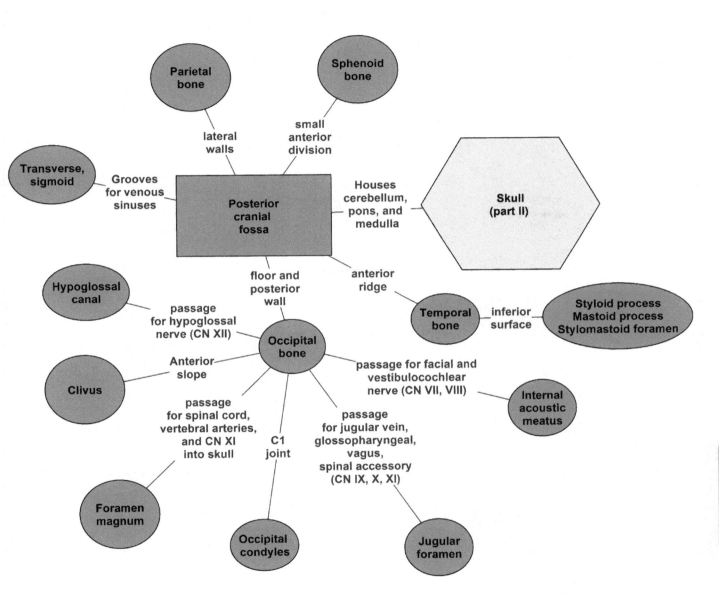

CM 5-5D

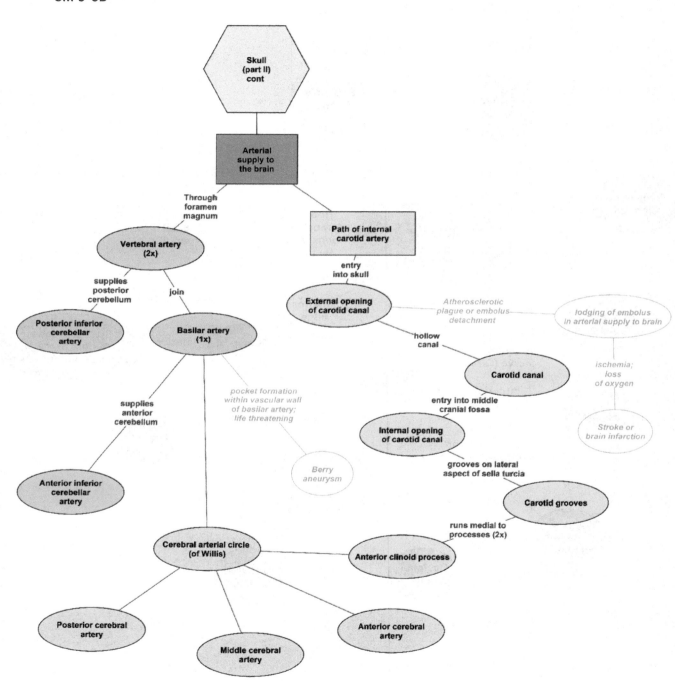

Synthesis Exercise: Create a concept map using items from EXERCISE 5-5A, 5-5B, 5-5C, and 5-5D.

Exercise 5-5A

Primary Category	Secondary Categories	Continuations
Skull- part II	Paranasal sinuses	Frontal sinus
	Anterior cranial fossa	Ethmoid sinus
		Sphenoidal sinus
		Maxillary sinus
		Frontal bone
		Ethmoid bone
		Sphenoid bone (3x)
		Orbital plate
		Cribiform plate
		Crista galli
		Anterior clinoid processes
		Lesser wing

Exercise 5-5B

Primary Category	Secondary Category	Continuations
Skull- part II	Middle cranial fossa	Greater wing
		Sphenoid body
		Temporal bone (2x)
		Superior orbital fissure
		Foramen spinosum
		Foramen ovale
		Foramen rotundum
		Optic canal
		Pre-chiasmatic groove
		Sella turcica
		Dorsum sellae
		Hypophysial fossa
		Tuberculum sellae
		Dorsum sellae
		Hypophysial fossa
		Tuberculum sellae
		Carotid groove
		Foramen lacerum

Primary Category	Secondary Category	Continuations
		Posterior clinoid processes
		Petrous part
		Squamous part
		Parietal bone

Exercise 5-5C

Primary Category	Secondary Category	Continuations
Skull- part II	Posterior cranial fossa	Transverse, sigmoid groove
		Occipital bone
		Hypoglossal canal
		Internal acoustic meatus
		Clivus
		Foramen magnum
		Jugular foramen
		Styloid process
		Mastoid process
		Stylomastoid foramen
		Occipital condyles

Exercise 5-5D

Primary Category	Secondary Categories	Continuations	Clinical Considerations
Skull- part II cont	Arterial supply to the brain	Path of internal carotid artery	Berry aneurysm
		Vertebral artery	Lodging of embolus in arterial supply to brain
		External opening of carotid canal	Stroke or brain infarction
		Posterior inferior cerebellar artery	
		Basilar artery	
		Anterior inferior cerebellar artery	
		Carotid canal	
		Internal opening of carotid canal	
		Carotid grooves	
		Anterior clinoid processes	
		Cerebral arterial circle (of Willis)	
		Posterior cerebral artery	
		Middle cerebral artery	
		Anterior cerebral artery	

VI. Hearing and Balance

Overview of key topics for this section:

- Anatomy of the ear
- Basis for hearing
- Basis for equilibrium and balance
- Acute otitis media
- Hearing loss
- Vertigo

What are the three divisions of the ear? How does the underlying anatomy mediate hearing? How does it mediate equilibrium?

Auditory sound is conveyed through three divisions of the ear: the external, middle, and inner ear. The **auricle**, or pinna, is part of the external ear and composed of auricular cartilage. It is quite flexible and functions to collect sound into the **external auditory canal**. The **helix** (outer) and **anti-helix** (inner) are two external rims of the auricle. The **tragus** (anterior) and **anti-tragus** (slightly posterior) are two ridges surrounding just the external acoustic meatus (or opening). The **concha** is a half loop leading into the external acoustic meatus. The remaining external ear contains the external auditory canal leading to the **tympanic membrane**. This thin membrane separates the external ear from the middle ear cavity (or tympanic cavity). In addition, its function is to vibrate in response to sound waves and convert the sounds waves into mechanical energy. The tympanic membrane oscillates to conducts sound to three small bones, collectively called ossicles: the **malleus**, the **incus**, and the **stapes**, which then transmit vibrations through the middle ear cavity. The base of the stapes is located on the **oval window** of the inner ear, and transmits the mechanical energy (oscillations) of the middle ear into pressure waves in the inner ear. The inner ear is embedded in the hollow **otic capsule** of the petrous ridge in the skull (the temporal bone). The bony labyrinth is a hollow space in the otic capsule filled with **perilymph**. The **membranous labyrinth** is within the bony labyrinth, suspended in the **perilymph**. The membranous labyrinth contains endolymph, which converts fluid waves to neural impulses.

Beginning at the **oval window**, the cochlea houses three ducts or canals,: the **scala vestibule** (or vestibular duct), filled with perilymph; the **scala tympani** (or tympanic duct), filled with perilymph; and the **scala media** (cochlear duct**), filled with endolymph. These ultimately convert pressure waves into electrical messages, called **action potentials**. The **cochlea** (a spiral cone; from Greek for snail) of the inner ear coils approximately 2.5 times and discontinues at an apex, called the **cupula**. As the base of the stapes vibrates within the oval window, pressure waves enter the scala vestibule and move toward the apex of the cochlea. High pitch sounds (i.e., high frequency sound waves) do not travel as far around the cochlea as low pitch sounds (i.e., low frequency sound waves). The pressure waves dissipate across the cochlear duct and initiate action potentials via mechanoreceptors, called hair cells, of the Organ of Corti (a spiral organ). Once initiated, action potentials are communicated to the brain via the cochlear branch of vestibulocochlear nerve (CN VIII). Finally, the pressure waves diffuse to the scala tympani and exit the cochlea via the **round window**. Thus, energy from the pressure waves are introduced into the oval window and leave through the round window. Furthermore, the distance traveled through the cochlea determines differences in pitch, according to a **tonotopic map**. For example, pressure waves from low pitch sounds travel a greater distance around the cochlear, whereas pressure waves from higher pitch sounds do not travel as far. An individual can interpret differences in pitch based on this principle, called tonotopic organization.

Equilibrium and balance of our bodies are determined within the **vestibular labyrinth** of the inner ear, comprised of the **vestibule**, in the center of the bony labyrinth, and three fluid-filled **semicircular canals,** each oriented in a different direction. The **utricle** and **saccule,** two small sacs filled with endolymph, contain specialized regions of mechanosensory epithelium, called **maculae**. The macula in the utricle is oriented in the horizontal plane, whereas the macula in the saccule is oriented in the vertical plane. During acceleration of the body, endolymph passes over the hair cells on the maculae to initiate action potentials. For example, riding in a car that is accelerating will initiate action potentials of the macula of the utricle due to its horizontal placement. Also, riding in an elevator that accelerates up and down will create action potential via the macula of the saccule due to its vertical placement. Action potentials are communicated to the brain via the vestibular branch of the vestibulocochlear nerve (CN VIII). Movements of the head (flexion, extension, rotation, and lateral bending) are perceived via the hair cells within the semicircular canals. Ampulla, or circular expansions, are found in each of the three semicircular canals. The horizontal, or lateral canal, responds to rotational movement (looking left and right) in the transverse plane. The superior or anterior canal is responsible for perceiving flexion and extension movements of the head (e.g., nodding) in the sagittal plane. The posterior canal tracks with lateral bending in the coronal plane. In addition to the utricle and saccule, movement of endolymph over specialized hair cells in each of the three ampulla allows the brain to determine the body's equilibrium and balance.

What is acute otitis media?

The middle ear cavity can become filled with fluid resulting from poor Eustachian tube function, which is relatively common early in life. The Eustachian tube connects the middle ear cavity with the nasopharynx. It serves to both equalize pressure of the middle ear and drain fluid into the **nasopharynx**. If the tube is not working properly due to allergies or bacterial infection, the middle ear can become inflamed leading to **acute otitis media**. Observing a swollen tympanic membrane with an otoscope can determine a diagnosis of acute otitis media. Antibiotic treatment is common, but it may also require a small incision of the tympanic membrane to relieve pressure and fluid buildup. A **myringotomy** tube may also supplement the incision to chronically drain the middle ear.

How does hearing loss occur?

Hearing loss can occur through three basic mechanisms including conductive hearing loss, sensory-neural hearing , and a combination of both. Complications with the transduction of mechanical energy within the outer and middle ear cavities can lead to conductive hearing loss. For example, several factors can promote conduction hearing loss, such as a buildup of ear wax in the auditory canal, excessive fluid inside the middle ear cavity, or injury to the tympanic membrane. Ultimately, this reduces the mechanical energy of the middle ear bones (the malleus, incus, and stapes) and leads to loss of hearing. A hearing aid can often help improve conductive hearing loss. A neural mechanism of hearing loss occurs via an inability to effectively receive or transmit sensory information to the brain. Causes may include destruction of hair cells due to excessive exposure to high volume sound, or compression of CN VIII via tumor growth. This type of hearing loss is more difficult to repair. Hearing loss may also include a combination of both conductive and sensory-neural.

What causes vertigo?

Dizziness or imbalance are symptoms of vertigo. This acute or chronic condition may originate from a variety of conditions. Motion sickness is an example of vertigo in which the brain received conflicting sensory input, such as riding in a car where you appear to be still, and looking out the window creating apparent motion. Special sensory input from the visual pathway (CN I) perceives movement of objects passing by while the vestibular special sensory (CN VIII) communicates little to no movement. Also, excessive alcohol consumption can dilute the endolymph of the inner ear and cause hyperactivity of special sensory hair cells. This can also lead to vertigo.

See CM 5-6A, 5-6B, and 5-6C for Review.

CM 5-6A

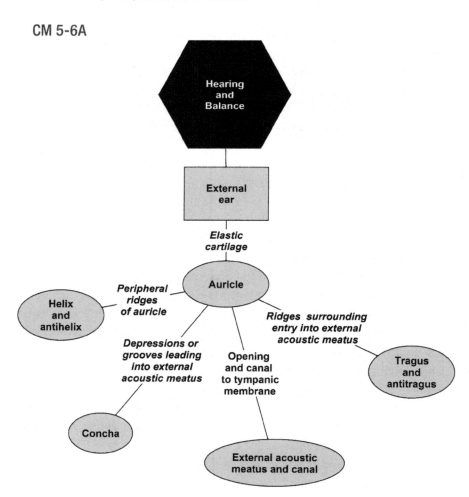

CM 5-6B

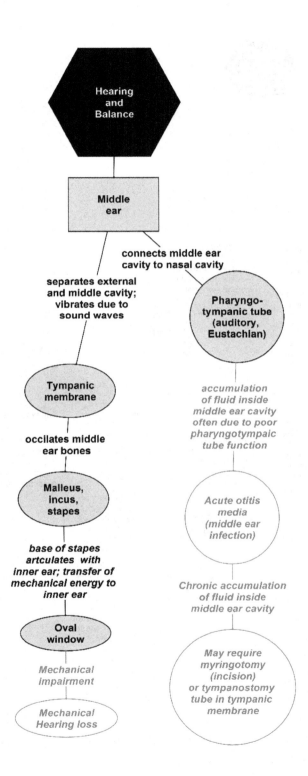

Hearing and Balance

Middle ear

connects middle ear cavity to nasal cavity

separates external and middle cavity; vibrates due to sound waves

Pharyngo-tympanic tube (auditory, Eustachian)

Tympanic membrane

accumulation of fluid inside middle ear cavity often due to poor pharyngotympaic tube function

occilates middle ear bones

Malleus, incus, stapes

Acute otitis media (middle ear infection)

base of stapes artculates with inner ear; transfer of mechanical energy to inner ear

Chronic accumulation of fluid inside middle ear cavity

Oval window

May require myringotomy (incision) or tympanostomy tube in tympanic membrane

Mechanical impairment

Mechanical Hearing loss

CHAPTER 5

CM 5-6C

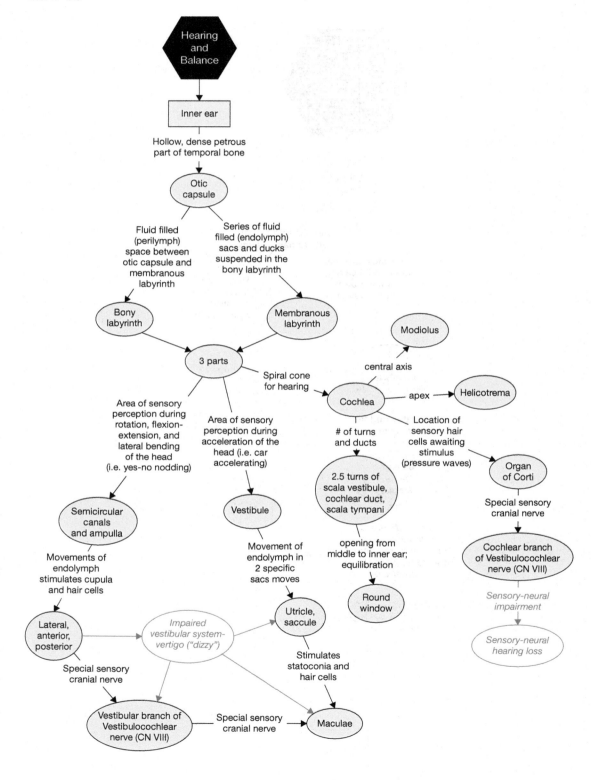

Synthesis Exercise: Create a concept map using items from EXERCISE 5-6A, 5-6B, and 5-6C.

Exercise 5-6A

Primary Category	Secondary Category	Continuations
Hearing and balance	External ear	Auricle
		Helix and antihelix
		External acoustic meatus and canal
		Tragus and antitragus
		Concha

Exercise 5-6B

Primary Category	Secondary Categor	Continuations	Clinical Considerations
Hearing and balance	Middle ear	Tympanic membrane	Mechanical hearing loss
		Otic capsule	Acute otitis media (middle ear infection)
		Pharyngotympanic tube	
		Bony labyrinth	May require myringotomy (incision) or tympanostomy tube in tympanic membrane
		Membranous labyrinth	
		Malleus, incus, stapes	
		Oval window	

Exercise 5-6C

Primary Category	Secondary Category	Continuations	Clinical Considerations
Hearing and balance	Inner ear	Otic capsule	Impaired vestibular system vertigo ("dizzy")
		Bony labyrinth	
		Membranous labyrinth	
		3 parts	
		Cochlea	
		Vestibule	
		Semicircular canals and ampulla	
		Modiolus	
		Helicotrema	
		Organ of Corti	
		2.5 turns of scala vestibule, cochlear duct, scala tympani	

Primary Category	Secondary Category	Continuations	Clinical Considerations
		Round window	
		Utricle, saccule	
		Lateral, anterior, posterior	
		Vestibular branch of Vestibulocochlear nerve (CN VIII)	
		Cochlear branch of Vestibulocochlear nerve (CN VIII)	

VII. Nasal Cavity, Oral Cavity, and Pharynx

Overview of key topics for this section:

- Nasal concha and meatus
- Nasal innervation and blood supply
- Tongue muscles and innervation
- Palate and arches
- Three divisions of the pharynx muscles and innervation

What is the nasal cavity? What are the nasal concha and meatus? What is the innervation and blood supply for the nasal cavity?

Deep to the nostrils (or naris), the **nasal cavity** lie on either side of the **nasal septum**. Part ethmoid (superior) and part vomer bone (inferior), the nasal septum divides the nasal cavity into a right and left side. On the lateral aspect of each nasal cavity are **nasal conchae** (or turbinates), which increase the surface area of the cavity and trap foreign debris from entering deep into the respiratory tract. These include three types called the superior, middle, and inferior nasal conchae. **Nasal meatuses** (superior, middle, and inferior) are located just inferior to the concha and include additional passageways to other areas of the facial region. For example, the **nasolacrimal duct** tracts from the medial orbit and drains near the inferior nasal meatus. The **Eustachian tube** from the middle ear cavity also drains posterior to the nasal cavity.

The arterial supply to the walls and septum of the nasal cavity include the **sphenopalatine artery** (originates at the maxillary) and **ethmoidal artery** (originates at the ophthalmic artery). Together, several arteries anastomose at **Kiesselbach's area,** which is a common site of nose bleed due to trauma or dry conditions. General sensory innervation to the nasal cavity occurs via the trigeminal nerve (CN V-0). Note that the upper half is V_1 (ophthalmic branch) and the lower half is V_2- (maxillary branch).

What are the four muscles of the tongue of the oral cavity? What innervates the muscles of the tongue and what are its actions? What innervates the surface of the tongue for general sensory and special sensory taste?

The **tongue** is a muscular structure in the oral cavity responsible for articulating speech and assisting in deglutition (or swallowing). It includes four specific muscles: the **genioglossus** for protrusion, the **hyoglossus** for depression, the **styloglossus** for elevation and retraction, and the **palatoglossus** for elevation of the posterior tongue. These muscles are innervated by the hypoglossal nerve (CN XII), except for the palatoglossus muscle, which is innervated by the vagus nerve (CN X) (see figure **5-7).**

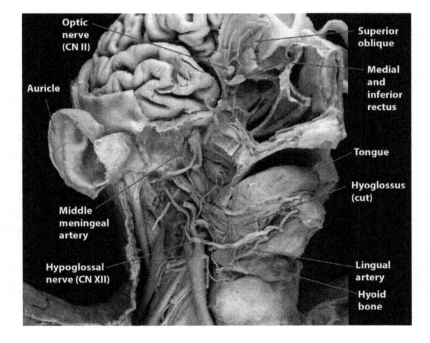

Figure 5-7

Optic nerve (CN II)

Superior oblique

Medial and inferior rectus

Auricle

Tongue

Hyoglossus (cut)

Middle meningeal artery

Hypoglossal nerve (CN XII)

Lingual artery

Hyoid bone

The surface of the tongue receives several innervations. The anterior two thirds is innervated by the **lingual nerve** of the trigeminal (CN V) for general sensory perception, like touch, temperature, and pain, and by the **chorda tympani** of the facial nerve (CN VII) to sense special tastes such as bitter, sweet, sour, etc. The posterior third of the tongue receives innervation for general sensory and special sensory taste through the glossopharyngeal nerve (CN IX). A small territory of the posterior third receives general and special sensory taste by the vagus nerve (CN X).

What functional deficits are included with damage to the hypoglossal nerve (CN XII)?

Following injury or lesioning of CN XII, a patient may experience disarticulation of speech (i.e., non-uniform speech) due to three of the four tongue muscles being affected. Also, if instructed to protrude the tongue (stick out the tongue), it will often deviate to the side of the hypoglossal nerve lesion. This is a result of a flaccid genioglossus tongue muscle on the side of the injury.

What muscles and other structures associate with the soft palate?

The **soft palate** (i.e., non-bone soft tissue), posterior to the palatine bone on the roof of oral cavity, is covered with mucosa. A cone-like projection called the **uvula** is attached to the soft palate. The **palatoglossus muscle, which** elevates the posterior tongue and **palatopharyngeus muscle**, which elevates the oral pharynx are muscles covered by mucosa. The **palatine tonsils**, made of lymphoid tissue and located between those two muscles, can become inflamed due to infection. This complex of muscles and tonsils are inferior to the soft palate, bilaterally. The **levator veli** and **levator veli palatini** are two additional muscles utilized during swallowing to elevate to elevate and tense the soft palate, respectively.. The palate (or roof of the mouth) is innervated for general sensory by the trigeminal nerve (V2 of CN V).

What is the pharynx and it's three divisions? What is its innervation?

The most superior aspect of the **pharynx,** is situated posterior to the nasal cavity and extends to the most inferior point lies just above the esophagus and larynx. Three divisions include the **nasopharynx** (posterior to the nasal cavity and above the soft palate), the **oropharynx** (posterior to the oral cavity, below the soft palate, and above the epiglottis), and the **laryngo-pharynx** (below the epiglottis and above the esophagus and larynx). The **pharyngeal constrictor muscles** (superior, middle, and inferior divisions) are primarily found on the posterior wall of the pharynx. Sensory innervation to the pharynx is via the glossopharyngeal nerve (CN XII) and motor innervation is through the vagus nerve (CN X). Both of these nerves work with the deglutition center in the medulla oblongata of the brain to coordinate swallowing.

See CM 5-7A, 5-7B, and 5-7C for Review.

CM 5-7A

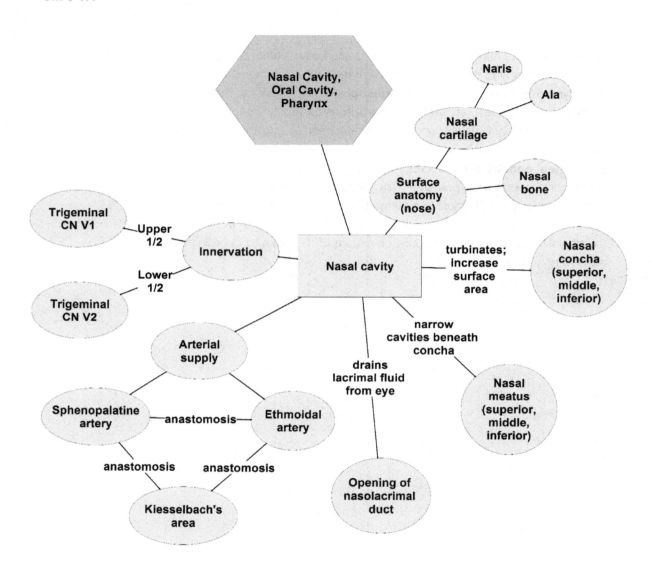

CM 5-7B

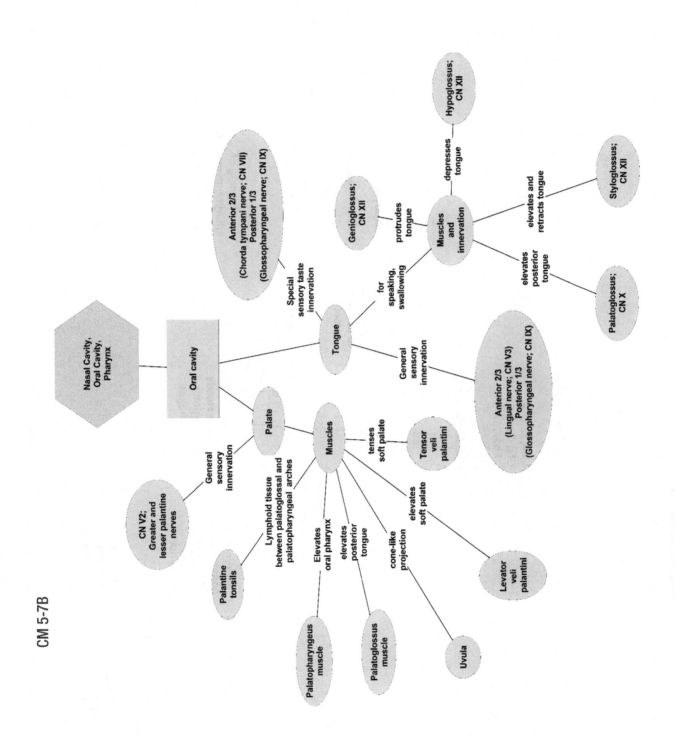

Nasal Cavity, Oral Cavity, Pharynx

Oral cavity

Tongue

Special sensory taste innervation

Anterior 2/3 (Chorda tympani nerve; CN VII) Posterior 1/3 (Glossopharyngeal nerve; CN IX)

for speaking, swallowing

Muscles and innervation

protrudes tongue

Genioglossus; CN XII

depresses tongue

Hypoglossus; CN XII

elevates and retracts tongue

Styloglossus; CN XII

elevates posterior tongue

Palatoglossus; CN X

General sensory innervation

Anterior 2/3 (Lingual nerve; CN V3) Posterior 1/3 (Glossopharyngeal nerve; CN IX)

Palate

General sensory innervation

CN V2; Greater and lesser palantine nerves

Lymphoid tissue between palatoglossal and palatopharyngeal arches

Palantine tonsils

Muscles

tenses soft palate

Tensor veli palantini

Elevates oral pharynx

Palatopharyngeus muscle

elevates posterior tongue

Palatoglossus muscle

cone-like projection

Uvula

elevates soft palate

Levator veli palantini

CM 5-7C

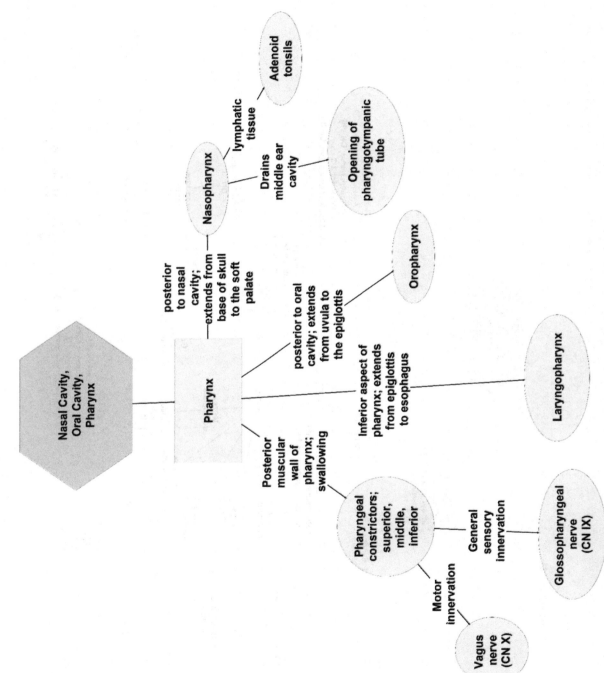

Nasal Cavity, Oral Cavity, Pharynx

Pharynx

posterior to nasal cavity; extends from base of skull to the soft palate

Nasopharynx

lymphatic tissue

Adenoid tonsils

Drains middle ear cavity

Opening of pharyngotympanic tube

posterior to oral cavity; extends from uvula to the epiglottis

Oropharynx

Inferior aspect of pharynx; extends from epiglottis to esophagus

Laryngopharynx

Posterior muscular wall of pharynx; swallowing

Pharyngeal constrictors; superior, middle, inferior

General sensory innervation

Glossopharyngeal nerve (CN IX)

Motor innervation

Vagus nerve (CN X)

Synthesis Exercise: Create a concept map using items from EXERCISE 5-7A, 5-7B, and 5-7C.

Exercise 5-7A

Primary Category	Secondary Category	Continuations
Nasal Cavity, Oral Cavity, Pharynx	Nasal cavity	Surface anatomy (nose)
		Nasal concha (superior, middle, inferior)
		Nasal meatus (superior, middle, inferior)
		Opening of nasolacrimal duct
		Arterial supply
		Ethmoidal artery
		Sphenopalatine artery
		Kiesselbach's area
		Innervation
		Trigeminal nerve (CN V2)
		Trigeminal nerve (CN V1)

Exercise 5-7B

Primary Category	Secondary Category	Continuations
Nasal Cavity, Oral Cavity, Pharynx	Oral cavity	Tongue
		Anterior 2/3 (chorda tympani; CN VII)
		Posterior 1/3 (Glossopharyngeal; CN IX)
		Anterior 2/3 (lingual nerve; CN V3)
		Posterior 1/3 (Glossopharyngeal; CN IX)
		Muscles and innervation
		Genioglossus; CN XII
		Hypoglossus; CN XII
		Styloglossus; CN XII
		Palatoglossus; CN X
		Palate
		Muscles
		Tensor veli palantini
		Levator veli palantini
		Uvuala
		Palatoglossus muscle
		Palatopharyngeus muscle
		Palantine tonsils
		Trigeminal CN V2; Greater and lesser palatine nerves

Exercise 5-7C

Primary Category	Secondary Category	Continuations
Nasal Cavity, Oral Cavity, Pharynx	Pharynx	Nasopharynx
		Oropharynx
		Laryngopharynx
		Adenoid tonsils
		Opening of pharyngotympanic tube
		Pharyngeal constrictors; superior, middle, inferior
		Vagus nerve CN X
		Glossopharyngeal nerve CN IX

VIII. Parasympathetics and Ganglion

Overview of key topics for this section:

- Oculomotor nerve (CN III) and the ciliary ganglion
- Glossopharyngeal nerve (CN IX) and the otic ganglion
- Facial nerve (CN VII) and the pterygopalatine ganglion
- Facial nerve (CN VII) and the submandibular ganglion

Which cranial nerve and associated ganglion is responsible for pupillary constriction via increased parasympathetic activity? Which nerve is associated with near versus distant vision?

In response to bright light or parasympathetic activation , the **oculomotor nerve** (CN III) increases parasympathetic neurons' presynaptic electrical impulses to the **ciliary ganglion**, where pre- and postsynaptic parasympathetic neurons synapse. Postsynaptic action potentials are carried to the posterior eyeball via short ciliary nerves. Depolarize **of sphincter pupillae muscles** cause contraction reducing the size of the pupil. This autonomic response helps prevent too much light from entering the eyeball (e.g., sunny day). Furthermore, postsynaptic sympathetic neurons innervate **dilator pupillae**

muscles to dilate the pupil, or increase its size, during a fight or flight response. This autonomic response also maximizes the entry of light into the eyeball.

In addition, ciliary muscles have parasympathetic innervation. These muscles help the zonular fibers of the lens relax and become more spherical in shape during near vision. Upon reduced parasympathetic innervation to the ciliary muscles, the zonular fibers create tension and the lens becomes flattened, for distant vision.

Which cranial nerve and associated ganglion is responsible for secretomotor input to the parotid gland via increased parasympathetic activity?

During parasympathetic activation (e.g., meal time), presynaptic neurons of the **glossopharyngeal nerve** (CN IX) transmit electrical impulses to the **otic ganglion** within the infratemporal fossa. Here, they synapse with postsynaptic parasympathetic neurons to communicate electrical impulses to the **parotid gland**. This salivary gland increases secretomotor activity (i.e., secretions) to release saliva into the parotid duct. The distal pathway of parotid gland innervation occurs via branches of the auriculotemporal nerve (mandibular nerve CN V_3) which house post-synaptic parasympathetic neurons . Coursing over the masseter muscle and piercing the buccinator muscle, the **parotid duct** delivers the newly secreted saliva into the oral cavity near the maxillary molar teeth. The saliva moistens food into a bolus and begins the digestive process. This autonomic response can occur prior to food being ingested into the oral cavity. Some of the special senses, such as vision and olfactory, can integrate with secretomotor activity of the parotid gland via CN IX.

Which cranial nerve and associated ganglion is responsible for secretomotor input to the lacrimal gland, nasal cavity, and palate via increased parasympathetic activity?

The pterygopalatine ganglion is located in the **pterygopalatine fossa**. This hollow region is found by entering the **pterygomaxillary fissure,** bound by the maxillary bone (anteriorly) and the lateral pterygoid plate (posteriorly). Within the pterygopalatine fossa are additional foramina, including the **foramen rotundum** or entry of the maxillary nerve (CN V_2), the **pterygoid**

canal for entry of the nerve to the pterygoid canal, the **sphenopalatine foramen,** for passage of sphenopalatine artery, and the **greater and lesser palatine canals,** for exit of the greater and lesser palatine nerves and arteries). During parasympathetic activation, presynaptic neurons from branches of the facial nerve (CN VII), called the **nerve to the pterygoid canal,** enter the pterygopalatine fossa via the pterygoid canal and synapse with postsynaptic parasympathetic neurons. Electrical impulses are then carried to the lacrimal gland via maxillary and zygomatic nerve branches (CN V2) and the lacrimal nerve (CN V1). This pathway increases secretomotor activity of the **lacrimal gland** to induce lacrimal fluid secretion over the eyeball. Emotional responses can also integrate with this pathway. Mucosal secretions in the nasal cavity and palate are activated similarly, except the post-synaptic parasympathetic neurons are destined for glands in the respective target tissues. However, the synapse still occurs in the pterygopalatine ganglion. In contrast, postsynaptic sympathetic neurons have opposite effects by reducing secretomotor activity to the mucosa of the nasal cavity and palate.

Which cranial nerve and associated ganglion are responsible for secretomotor to the submandibular and sublingual gland via increased parasympathetic activity?

The **submandibular ganglion,** located superior to the deep portion of the **submandibular gland**, is where the pre- and postsynaptic neurons synapse, leading to increased salivation during parasympathetic activation. The **chorda tympani** branch of the facial nerve (CN VII) meets with the lingual nerve of CN V3 and transmits electrical impulses to the submandibular ganglion (presynaptic). Postsynaptic glandular nerves are responsible for secretomotor innervation to both the submandibular and sublingual gland. This pathway leads to increased salivation within the oral cavity during rest and digest conditions.

See CM 5-8A for Review.

CM 5-8A

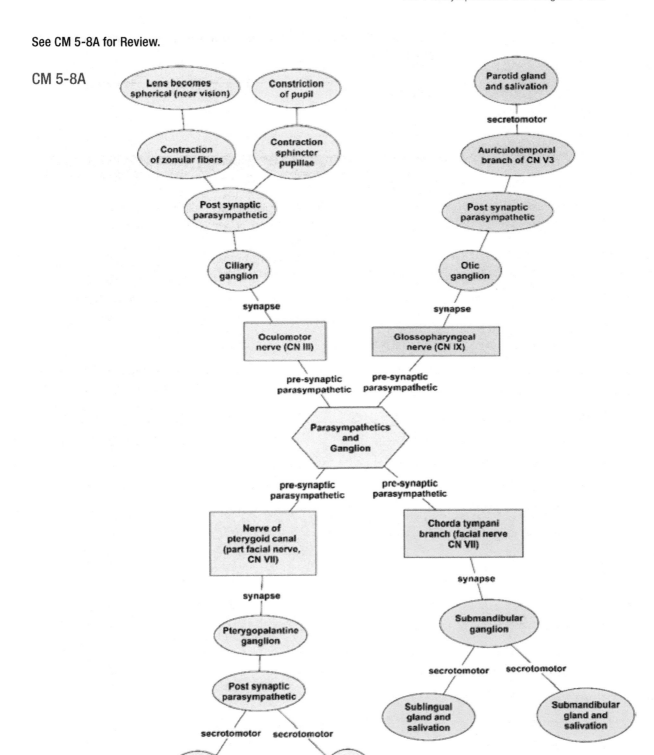

Synthesis Exercise: Create a concept map using items from EXERCISE 5-8.

Exercise 5-8

Primary Category	Secondary Categories	Continuations
Parasympathetics and ganglion	Oculomotor CN III	Ciliary ganglion
	Glossopharyngeal CN IX	Otic ganglion
	Chorda tympanic branch of facial nerve CN VII	Pterygopalatine ganglion
	Nerve of pterygoid canal (part facial nerve CN VII)	Submandibular ganglion
		Post synaptic parasympathetic (4x)
		Contraction of sphincter pupillae
		Contraction of zonular fibers
		Auriculotemporal branch of CN V3
		Parotid gland and salivation
		Lens becomes spherical (near vision)
		Constriction of pupil
		Nasal cavity glands
		Palatine glands
		Sublingual gland and salivation
		Submandibular gland and salivation

Image Credits

- Fig. 5-1: Copyright © 2016 by 4D Anatomy. Reprinted with permission.
- Fig. 5-2: Copyright © 2016 by 4D Anatomy. Reprinted with permission.
- Fig. 5-3: Copyright © 2016 by 4D Anatomy. Reprinted with permission.
- Fig. 5-4: Copyright © 2016 by 4D Anatomy. Reprinted with permission.
- Fig. 5-5: Copyright © 2016 by 4D Anatomy. Reprinted with permission.
- Fig. 5-6: Copyright © 2016 by 4D Anatomy. Reprinted with permission.
- Fig. 5-7: Copyright © 2016 by 4D Anatomy. Reprinted with permission.

Chapter 6
Thorax

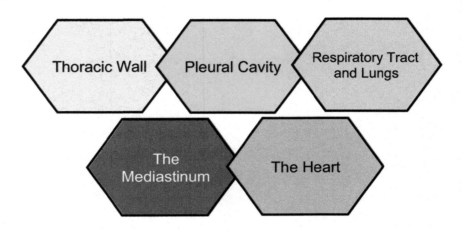

Overview of the Thorax

The thorax, located between the neck and the abdomen, houses the lungs, heart, major vessels of the mediastinum, esophagus, thoracic duct, trachea, and distal respiratory tract. Breast tissue houses the mammary glands within the subcutaneous fascia of the thorax. The thoracic wall, composed of ribs, costal cartilage, sternum, and thoracic vertebrae (back region), provide the majority of protection in this region. A variety of surface anatomy landmarks allows for navigation of the underlying mediastinum and pleural cavities. The cardiopulmonary system (i.e., heart and lungs) promotes re-oxygenation of blood through a tightly coupled and dynamic process of ventilation.

I. Thoracic Wall and Associated Structures

Overview of key topics for this section:

- Basic structure and function
- Surface landmarks of the thoracic wall
- Superior and inferior thoracic apertures
- Osteology of the thoracic wall
- Intercostal space, muscles, and neurovasculature
- Intercostal nerve block
- Ideal gas law and ventilation
- The diaphragm
- Hemidiaphragmatic paralysis
- Mechanisms of quiet versus deep ventilation
- Introduction to the breast tissue
- Breast cancer metastasis
- Note: See Chapter 3 for pectoralis, serratus anterior, and subclavius muscles

What is the thoracic wall? Basic structure? Basic function?

The **thoracic wall** is composed of ribs, sternum, costal cartilage, intercostal muscles, superficial muscles, subcutaneous fascia, and overlying skin in the region **(see figure 6-1)**. The posterior aspect includes the vertebrae, which are technically considered part of the back region. In addition to protection of the underlying heart, lungs, and major vessels, the thoracic wall maintains space for the lungs (i.e., **pleural cavities**) and assist with ventilation. It also supports the attachment of the upper limb via the pectoral girdle (clavicle and scapula).

Where are the surface anatomy landmarks of the thorax?

Navigating the thoracic region requires several key surface anatomy landmarks. In the anterior thoracic wall, the **suprasternal notch** (or jugular

Figure 6-1

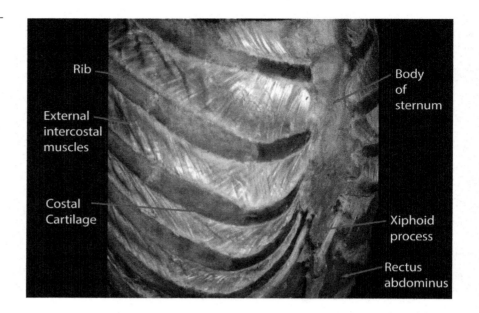

notch; T2 vertebra level) is found at the superior aspect of the manubrium. Between the inferior border of the manubrium and the superior aspect of the sternal body is the **sternal angle** (intervertebral disc of T4, T5). At the **xiphisternal junction** (T9 vertebra level), an articulation occurs between the inferior part of the manubrium body and the xiphoid process of the sternum. The **xiphoid process** of the sternum is found at the T10 vertebra level. The most inferior aspect of the thoracic cage, the **costal margin,** serves as an attachment site for the diaphragm.

Several surface anatomy lines in the vertical direction are also helpful when describing specific locations in the thoracic region. The **anterior median line** is within the median plane (midline) and the **parasternal lines** are located on the lateral most aspect of the sternum. The **midclavicular lines** course vertically through the midpoint of the clavicle. On the lateral aspect of the thorax are the **axillary lines** which include the anterior axillary (i.e., pectoral fold), mid-axillary (i.e., middle), and posterior axillary (i.e., latissimus dorsi fold) lines. The **posterior median line** is in the median plane (midline) on the posterior thoracic wall and the **paravertebral lines** align vertically with the transverse processes of the vertebrae. **Scapular lines** align vertically with the inferior angle of the scapula.

Where are the superior and inferior thoracic apertures? What major structures pass through the apertures? What are the respective vertebral levels? What is a hiatal hernia?

The **superior thoracic aperture** represents a transition from the thorax to the neck. It is an opening in the most superior aspect of the thoracic cage, produced by the manubrium (anteriorly), the first ribs (laterally), and the T1 vertebra (posteriorly). Contents passing through the superior thoracic aperture include the trachea, esophagus, apex of the lungs, nerves, and major blood vessels. The **inferior thoracic aperture** is found at the costal margin. Although the diaphragm attaches to the costal margin, the abdominal viscera push it superiorly into the thorax. Thus, the diaphragm, and not the inferior thoracic aperture, designate the true transition from the thorax to the abdomen. Furthermore, the diaphragm has three specific passageways (i.e., apertures) between the thorax and abdomen. At the T8 vertebra level, the **caval foramen** allows the inferior vena cava (IVC) and right phrenic nerve to pass through. The **esophageal hiatus** at the T10 vertebra level includes a passageway for the esophagus, the vagus nerves, and some esophageal vessels. The superior aspect of the stomach can potentially herniate through the esophageal hiatus into the thorax. This condition is called a **hiatal hernia** and may occur due to a weakening in the muscular diaphragm tissue at this location. Obesity is a risk factor for hiatal hernias. At the T12 vertebra level, the **aortic hiatus** allows the aorta and thoracic duct to course through the diaphragm.

What forms the skeleton of the thoracic wall? What dynamic joints are present?

The skeleton of the thoracic wall includes the ribs, sternum, and costal cartilage. Additionally, the thoracic vertebrae of the back support the posterior aspect of the thorax. The ribs articulate with, and extend from, the thoracic vertebrae in an anterior and inferior direction. Thus, the ribs are tilted forward and not horizontal. On each side, 12 ribs typically exist. A skeleton had three types of ribs: **true ribs** (1–7), which have individual costal cartilage associated with the sternum, **false ribs** (8–10), which share a **costal arch**, and **floating ribs** (11–12), which do not attach to costal cartilage. Aberrant cervical ribs are rare but can articulate with, and extend from, the lower cervical vertebrae. A typical rib includes a head with two facets (superior, inferior) for articulating with the vertebra above and below called a **costovertebral joint**. The superior facet of the rib articulates with the **inferior costal facet** of the vertebra above. Similarly, the inferior facet articulates with the **superior costal facet** of the vertebra below. Together, the superior and inferior costal facets are called the **demifacets**. The neck of the rib is located between the head and the tubercle. A facet of the tubercle articulates with the transverse process of the same number as the rib, called a **costotransverse joint** (i.e rib 7 articulates with transverse process of T7 vertebra). Both the costovertebral and costotransverse joints allow for rotation (e.g., elevation, depression) via an axis through the head and neck of the rib. The **costal angle** of the rib is a sharp curvature that measuring about one third the length from the head of the rib. A **costal groove,** located along the inferior surface of the length of the rib, serves to protect the neurovasculature of the intercostal space. An articulation between the anterior end of the rib and the costal cartilage is called the **costochondral joint**. A **sternocostal joint** is located between the costal cartilage and the sternum. The sternum is located in the anterior thoracic wall and divided into the three parts. The shape of the sternum is characterized much like a sword. The **manubrium** (handle of the sword) is the most superior aspect and articulates with the **body of the manubrium** (shaft of the sword). At the most inferior aspect of the manubrium is the xiphoid process (tip of the sword).

Where is the intercostal space? What muscles are located here and what is its function? What is its innervation? What bundle or neurovasculature resides in the intercostal space? What other muscles assist the thoracic wall and do not reside within the intercostal space?

The **intercostal space** is located between two adjacent ribs (superior and inferior ribs). On each side, 12 ribs are present, creating 11 intercostal spaces. Several types of muscle groups reside within the intercostal space, including the external intercostal, internal intercostal, and the innermost intercostal. The **external intercostal muscle** is most active during forced inspiration (e.g., rigorous exercise), and functions to elevate the thoracic cage (discussed in more detail later). Muscle fibers in this group are oriented anteriorly and inferiorly (like your hands and fingers in your pockets). Deep to the external intercostal muscle, the **internal intercostal muscles** participate in forced exhalation, functioning to compress the thoracic cage. Muscle fibers are directed anteriorly and superiorly (like your hands and fingers on your chest; uncrossed and pointed superiorly). The external intercostal muscles are not present in the anterior aspect of the thoracic wall, but rather, continuous as an aponeurosis. Similarly, the internal intercostal muscles are absent posteriorly and replaced by a membrane. A third and even deeper group, called the **innermost intercostals,** is a not a true muscle group. However, it can be delicately separated from the overlying internal intercostal muscles. Between the internal intercostal and innermost group, a neurovascular bundle occupies each intercostal space. The primary bundle runs within the costal groove of the superior rib while collateral (secondary) branches course just above the inferior rib. Each intercostal bundle contains a vein, artery, and nerve. A helpful learning aid is to remember the sequence of structures in V.A.N. from superior to inferior. **Intercostal nerves** from anterior rami of T1–T11 provide innervation to the intercostal muscles. Also, lateral and anterior branches spread over the respective regions of the thoracic wall for cutaneous innervation. Pleural branches of the intercostal nerve help innervate the parietal pleura of the lungs. Intercostal nerves T7–T11 continue across the subcostal margin to supply the anterolateral abdominal wall and are considered **thoracoabdominal nerves**. The anterior **intercostal arteries,** which arise from the **internal thoracic artery (**bilaterally; originating from the subclavian artery), supply the anterior third of the thoracic wall. The posterior intercostal arteries supply the posterior two thirds of the thoracic wall and originate from the aorta. An anastomosis occurs between the anterior and posterior intercostal arteries. The internal thoracic artery bifurcates to the **musculophrenic artery** (to supply to intercostal spaces 7–9) and the **superior epigastric artery** (to supply part of the diaphragm and rectus abdominis muscle). The posterior **intercostal veins** drain into the azygos venous system (posteriorly), the internal thoracic veins (anteriorly), and the brachiocephalic veins **(see figure 6-2)** Four to six **transverse thoracic muscles,** deep and anterior on each side of the thoracic wall, attach from the sternum to the costal cartilage. Their proposed function is to compress the thoracic cage. The **subcostal muscles** on the very deep aspect of the thoracic wall typically span two intercostal segments.

Figure 6-2

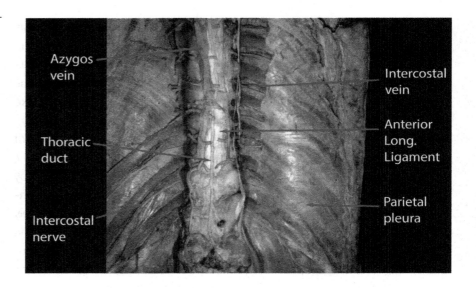

Azygos vein

Thoracic duct

Intercostal nerve

Intercostal vein

Anterior Long. Ligament

Parietal pleura

What is an intercostal nerve block?

Patients with an inflamed or irritated intercostal nerve may require an **intercostal nerve block** for relief. Herpes zoster virus or chest surgery may exacerbate the inflammation. A needle is directed in the affected intercostal space near the superior aspect (primary intercostal nerve) and inferior aspect (collateral or secondary intercostal nerve) via 2 separate injections. Steroid injections are a common pharmacologic tool to provide acute pain relief. Technical expertise and close attention to the location of the intercostal nerves help prevent direct damage to the nerve during the injection.

What is Boyle's law (the ideal gas law)? How does it translate ventilation in humans?

Ventilation is a mechanism for breathing (i.e., inhalation and exhalation) based on principles of **Boyle's law (or the ideal gas law)**. Boyle's law ($PV=nRT$) states that if temperature and volume of gas remain constant, then volume and pressure are inversely related. Thus, if volume of a closed system decreases, then pressure increases. And vice versa, if volume increases, then pressure decreases. Pulmonary ventilation responds primarily to the action of the diaphragm. During inhalation, the diaphragm contracts and pushes the abdominal viscera (liver) inferiorly. This promotes (1) increased volume of the pleural cavity and lungs, (2) decreased pressure in the pleural cavity and lungs as compared to the atmosphere, and (3) negative pressure drawing air into the lungs. During exhalation, the diaphragm relaxes and the abdominal viscera (liver) push superiorly. This promotes: (1) decreased volume of the pleural cavity and lungs, (2) increased pressure in the pleural cavity and lungs as compared to the atmosphere, and (3) positive pressure pushing air out of the lungs.

What is the diaphragm?

The **diaphragm** is the primary skeletal muscle responsible for ventilation, or breathing. It is innervated by the **phrenic nerve** (originates at C3, C4, C5 spinal nerves). Proximal attachments of the diaphragm include the **xiphoid process**, **costal margin**, the lower ribs, and T1–L2 vertebrae. A **right and left crus** (tendinous structures) support the posterior attachment to the vertebrae and also creates a hiatus for the aorta. The distal attachment is the **central tendon** or a tough aponeurosis. When relaxed, the diaphragm is pushed superiorly, and assumes a right and left dome shape. During contraction, the diaphragm pushes inferiorly and becomes flattened. The **pericardial sac** of the heart fuses with the central tendon of the diaphragm, allowing the apex of the heart to move inferiorly and promote a more vertical position when the diaphragm contracts. Thus, the positioning of the heart is not completely static. The arterial supply is the **pericardiacophrenic** (originates from the internal thoracic artery), **musculophrenic** (originates from the internal thoracic artery), and **inferior phrenic arteries** (originates from abdominal aorta). The diaphragm represents a divide between the thorax and the abdomen.

What is hemidiaphragmatic paralysis?

Damage to the phrenic nerve, cervical spinal region, or the brain stem can cause the dysfunction in the diaphragm. For example, a lesion (or cut) to the right phrenic nerve , causes the right side of the diaphragm (ipsilateral) to remain dome shape and more superior than the left diaphragm (contralateral) during contraction. This effect is known as **hemidiaphragmatic paralysis.** It can be observed via imaging, such as radiography. Although ventilation can still occur on the ipsilateral side, overall respiratory capacity is significantly reduced.

What are the mechanisms of quiet breathing? Deep ventilation?

A normal respiratory rate (inhalation, exhalation) at rest for adults is 12–18 cycles per min. At younger ages, the range can be high as 40 cycles per minute, as in newborns. **Quiet breathing** occurs during non-stressed and sedentary behavior. The primary muscle that facilitates quiet breathing is the diaphragm.

During intense exercise or a true sympathetic response (e.g., fight or flight), the respiratory rate can range from 40–50 cycles per minute in adults. The respiratory capacity (or volume of air exchanged) increases in this situation and is often referred to as **deep ventilation** (forced inspiration, forced exhalation). During forced inhalation, the **pump handle mechanism** increases the anterior-to-posterior diameter of the thoracic cavity following contraction of the external intercostal muscles. Secondly, the **bucket handle mechanism** increases the transverse diameter of the thoracic cavity via contraction of the external intercostal muscles. In contrast to the external intercostals, the internal intercostals help depress the thorax in the anterior-to-posterior and transverse directions during forced expiration During deep ventilation, movements at the costovertebral, costotransverse, sternocostal, and interchondral joints facilitate these types of movements.

Where is the breast tissue?

Breast tissue is found subcutaneously on the anterior thoracic wall in both females and males. Both sexes have bilateral nipples surrounded by an areola on the surface of the skin. In females, 15–20 **mammary gland lobules** per breast produce breast milk for newborns. Breast milk travels through the mammary gland to the **lactiferous duct** and to **lactiferous sinuses** just deep to the nipple. Hormones (prolactin, oxytocin, estrogen, progesterone) control the production of milk and its release, referred to as the let-down reflex, and mechanical stimulation of the nipple. **Suspensory ligaments (Cooper's ligaments)** and adipose help support the breast tissue. The **lateral thoracic artery** (originates from the axillary artery) and the **medial mammary arteries** (originates from the internal thoracic artery) supply the respective regions of the breast. Subscapular, pectoral, and parasternal lymph nodes help drain lymph fluid from the breast into the general circulation. Males typically have remnants of mammary glands, which remain underdeveloped due to lack of hormonal influence.

What is breast cancer metastasis?

Breast cancer can promote dimpling of the skin due to invasion of the suspensory ligaments. Breast cancer cells can also metastasize (i.e., move to and invade additional alternative tissue sites) through lymphatic drainage. A biopsy of the lymph nodes can determine the stage of breast cancer development, which assists with therapeutic strategies. A **mastectomy** is the surgical removal of breast tissue due to cancer development.

See CM 6-1A and 6-1B for review.

CM 6-1A

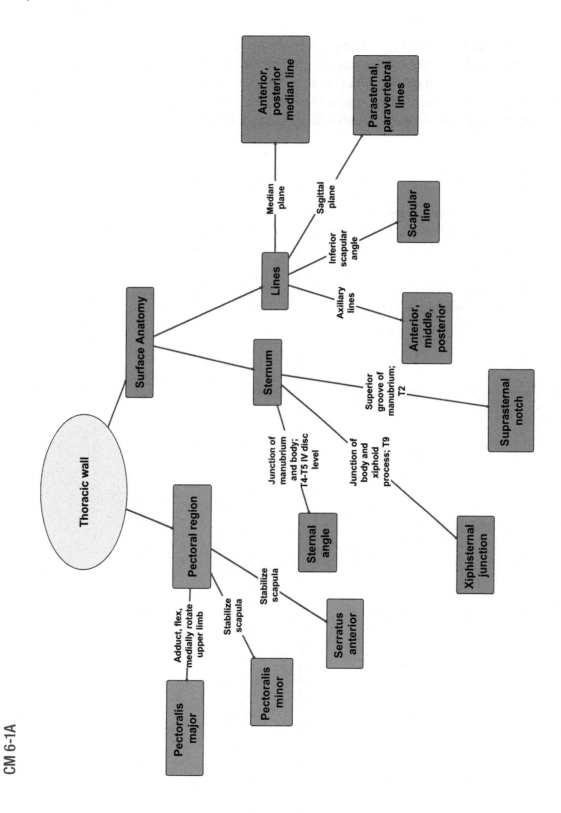

Thoracic wall

Surface Anatomy

Pectoral region

- Pectoralis major — Adduct, flex, medially rotate upper limb
- Pectoralis minor — Stabilize scapula
- Serratus anterior — Stabilize scapula

Lines
- Anterior, posterior median line — Median plane
- Parasternal, paravertebral lines — Sagittal plane
- Scapular line — Inferior scapular angle
- Anterior, middle, posterior — Axillary lines

Sternum
- Suprasternal notch — Superior groove of manubrium; T2
- Sternal angle — Junction of manubrium and body; T4-T5 IV disc level
- Xiphisternal junction — Junction of body and xiphoid process; T9

CM 6-1B

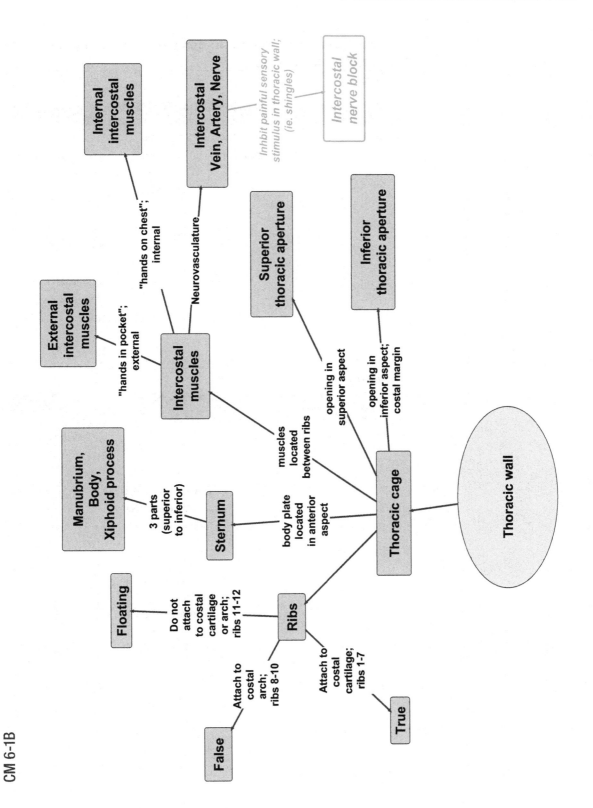

Synthesis Exercise: Create a concept map using items from EXERCISE 6-1A and 6-1B.

Exercise 6-1A

Primary Category	Secondary Categories	Continuations
Thoracic Wall	Surface anatomy	Lines
	Pectoral region	Sternum
		Serratus anterior
		Pectoralis minor
		Pectoralis major
		Anterior, posterior median line
		Parasternal, paravertebral line
		Scapular line
		Anterior, middle, posterior line
		Suprasternal notch
		Xiphisternal junction

Exercise 6-1B

Primary Category	Secondary Categories	Continuations	Clinical Considerations
Thoracic Wall	Thoracic cage	Ribs	Intercostal nerve block
		Sternum	
		Intercostal muscles	
		Superior thoracic aperture	
		Inferior thoracic aperture	
		True	
		False	
		Floating	
		Manubrium, body, xiphoid process	
		External intercostal muscles	
		Internal intercostal muscles	
		Intercostal vein, artery, nerve	

II. Pleural Cavity

Overview of key topics for this section:

- Pleural cavities and pleural linings
- Pleural reflections and recesses
- Pneumothorax and Hemothorax
- Thoracocentesis

Where are the pleural cavities? What are the pleural linings? Parietal versus visceral?

The lungs and pleural linings are located inside the **pleural cavities**, a hollow region inside the thorax on either side of the mediastinum. The right and left pleural cavities are separate and completely isolated from each other. On the deep aspect of the thoracic wall is **endothoracic fascia** (glue-like material) which adheres the **parietal pleura** (similar to wallpaper) of the lungs **(see figure 6-2)**. In addition to its attachment to the deep thoracic wall, the parietal pleura surround the lungs in each of the respective pleural cavities. The parietal pleura is named for its respective location in relation to the lung: (1) the costal (lateral, anterior, posterior); (2) mediastinal (medial); (3) diaphragmatic (inferior); and (4) cervical (superior) parietal pleura. The main bronchi , pulmonary artery (supplies deoxygenated blood), and pulmonary veins (drains oxygenated blood) enter the lung on the mediastinal (medial) surface at the **hilum of the lung**. It is here that the parietal pleura is continuous with and transitions into the **visceral pleura** of the lung. The visceral pleura adheres closely to the lung and cannot be separated from its surface. Taken together, the parietal and visceral pleura represent a sac (or a collapsed balloon) and the lungs have invaginated into the pleural sac. Between the parietal and visceral pleura is **pleural fluid,** which promotes surface tension between these two pleural layers. Functionally, the pleural fluid allows free movement (inflation and deflation) of the lung in response to changes of intrathoracic pressure. The parietal pleura is innervated by branches of the phrenic and intercostal nerves. **Pleurisy** is a condition whereby the pleura becomes inflamed.

What are the pleural reflections and recesses?

The parietal pleura changes its direction as it passes from one wall of the thoracic cavity to another. These specific sites along the wall are named lines of pleural reflection. For example, at the anterior junction of the costal pleura and mediastinal pleura is the **sternal line of pleural reflection**. At the posterior junction of the costal pleura and mediastinal pleura is the **vertebral line of pleural reflection.** Inferiorly, the junction of the costal pleura with the diaphragmatic pleura is called the **costal line of pleural reflection**.

Pleural recesses are formed as potential spaces, and are not filled with lung tissue during normal breathing. For example, the costal pleura and the diaphragmatic pleura contact each other in the **costodiaphragmatic recess** following exhalation. However, during deep inhalation this potential space temporarily converts into a real space which fills the recess with lung tissue. The real space of the costodiaphragmatic recess is converted back into a potential space upon exhalation. A second type of a pleural recess is the **costomediastinal recess,** formed by contact between the costal and mediastinal pleurae. Although smaller in size compared to the costodiaphragmatic recess, it also converts from a potential space to a real space. The left **costomediastinal recess** is larger than the right due to the cardiac notch (less occupied).

What is a pneumothorax (one way versus two way)? What is a hemothorax?

Following a puncture wound to the thorax (e.g., bullet or knife trauma), a pneumothorax may develop and the lung will likely collapse. The introduction of air into the pleural cavity removes surface tension between the parietal pleura and visceral pleura. In this setting, the lung recoils and lacks the ability to inflate. In a **one-way pneumothorax**, air travels directly from the atmosphere into the pleural cavity, but cannot travel outward due to the unidirectional flap of tissue. Thus, air pressure inside the pleural cavity increases on the ipsilateral side (same side as the injury) and potentially impedes the contralateral pleural cavity (side opposite the injury). Unless the pressure is equalized via an emergency chest tube, the contralateral lung is at risk for compression and dysfunction. In a two-way pneumothorax, atmospheric air travels directly into the pleural cavity and can also escape outward. The tissue flap in this setting is bidirectional. Emergency clinical care may attempt to cover the two-way pneumothorax to prevent air from entering the pleural cavity. Similarly, a hemothorax occurs when blood accumulates inside the pleural cavity due to trauma to the thorax (e.g., laceration of the lung or artery, such as the internal thoracic artery). In this situation, the blood separates the parietal and visceral pleurae of the lung. Also, blood typically collects in the costodiaphragmatic recess if a patient is upright. Either thoracostomy drainage via a tube or thoracocentesis can treat a hemothorax.

What is a thoracocentesis?

A thoracocentesis, or pleural tap, is a procedure that uses a syringe and needle to remove fluid accumulated in the pleural cavity. The patient assumes an upright position to accumulate fluid in the costodiaphragmatic recess. Sources may vary with regard to the site of needle placement, but effectiveness has been shown in the mid-axillary line ranging from the 6th–9th intercostal space. Importantly, the clinician uses technical expertise to avoid puncturing the lungs.

See CM 6-2A for Review.

CM 6-2A

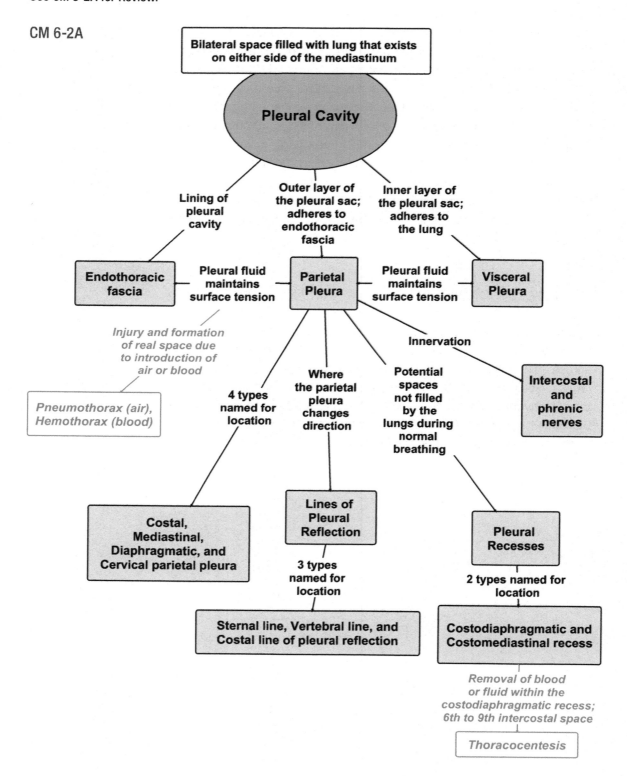

Synthesis Exercise: Create a concept map using items from EXERCISE 6-2.

Exercise 6-2

Primary Category	Secondary Categories	Continuations	Clinical Considerations
Pleural Cavity	Endothoracic Fascia Parietal Pleura Visceral Pleura	Intercostal and phrenic nerves Pleural recesses Lines of pleural reflection Costal, mediastinal, diaphragmatic, and cervical parietal pleura Costodiaphragmatic and costomediastinal recess Sternal line, vertebral line, and costal line of pleural reflection	Thoracocentesis Pneumothorax (air) Hemothorax (blood)

III. The Respiratory Tract and Lungs

Overview of key topics for this section:

- Trachea and main bronchi
- Hilum of the lungs
- Major nerves in the region
- Lobes and surfaces of the lung
- Brochopulmonary segments
- Surgical resection of the lungs
- Bronchioles and alveolar sacs
- Pulmonary circulation
- Ductus arteriosum and ligamentum arteriosum
- Pulmonary embolism
- Lymph drainage

What is the trachea? What is the hilum of the lungs? What are the respective vertebral levels for the trachea? Where does the trachea transition to the right and left main bronchi?

The **trachea** is located at the inferior aspect of the cricoid cartilage of the larynx at approximately the C6 vertebral level. This cartilaginous tube provides a passageway for air between the larynx and the main bronchi. It is approximately 10–16 cm long (4–6 in) and about 25 cm (1 in) in diameter. Several cartilaginous rings keep the trachea patent (open). At the **carina,** located at approximately the T4/T5 intervertebral disc and the sternal angle (or transverse thoracic plane), the trachea bifurcates into the right and left main bronchi. The right main bronchus is wider and more vertical relative to the left main bronchus. Thus, an inhaled foreign object (e.g., food or small object) typically lodges in the right main bronchus more often than the left. The main bronchi enter the lung tissue with the pulmonary artery and pulmonary veins at the **hilum,** or root of the lung.

What major nerves reside in this region?

The hilum of the lungs facilitates identification of the **phrenic** and **vagus** nerves. The phrenic nerve is courses anterior to the hilum and the vagus nerve remains posterior to the hilum. In addition, the sympathetic and parasympathetic nervous systems participate in the **pulmonary plexus**, a network of nervous tissue, which communicates changes in bronchiole diameter (respiratory tissue) and vascular diameter (non-respiratory tissue). Smooth muscle contraction and relaxation enables such changes (dilation and constriction).

What are the lobes of the right and left lungs? What are the fissures? What are the surfaces of the lungs? What respiratory and vascular structures supply each lobe of the lung?

The right and left lungs are similar, yet have specific differences. The right lung has a superior, a middle, and an inferior lobe. A **horizontal fissure** separates the superior and middle lobe, and the **oblique fissure** (at an angle) divides the middle from the inferior lobe. The left lung has only a superior and an inferior lobe, which are separated by the oblique fissure. the most inferior-anterior aspect of the superior lobe of the left lung has a tongue-like feature, called the **lingula**. Just superior is the **cardia notch**, a slight curvature of the superior lobe created by the impression of the heart. Each lung has several surfaces labeled the **costal surface,** associated with the ribs; the **diaphragmatic surface** at the inferior aspect; and the **mediastinal surface** medially. Each lung also has three ridge-like borders. The anterior border is the junction of the anterior costal and anterior mediastinal surfaces; the posterior border represents the junction of the posterior costal and posterior mediastinal surfaces; and the inferior border is the transition from both the costal and mediastinal surfaces to the diaphragmatic surface. Each main bronchi divides into **secondary,** or **lobar bronchi,** which correspond to the lobes of each lung: right a superior, middle, and inferior lobar bronchus for the right lung, and a superior and inferior lobar bronchus for the left lung. Similarly, lobar arteries and veins accompany the lobar bronchi.

What are the bronchopulmonary segments of the right and left lungs? What respiratory and vascular structures supply the bronchopulmonary segment of the lung?

The lobes of the lungs are further subdivided into **brochopulmonary segments**. Each segment is supplied by **tertiary or segmental bronchi and** segmental arteries and veins.

Bronchopulmonary Segments

- Right lung: ten brochopulomnary segments:
    - *Superior lobe segments*
        1 apical
        2 posterior
        3 anterior
    - *Middle lobe segments*
        1 lateral
        2 medial

- *Inferior lobe segments-*
  1 superior
  2 anterior basal
  3 medial basal
  4 lateral basal
  5 posterior basal

- Left lung: eight bronchopulomnary segments, some of which are typically combined:
  - *Superior lobe segments*
    1 apicoposterior (apical and posterior combined)
    2 anterior
    3 lingular (superior and inferior combined)
  - *Inferior lobe segments*
    1 superior
    2 anterior basal
    3 medial basal
    4 lateral basal
    5 posterior basal

Where can the lung be surgically resected?

Lung cancer patients may require the surgical resection, or removal, of lung tissue. For example, a **pneumonectomy** removes an entire lung through open chest surgery, referred to as a **thoracotomy**. If a smaller portion of the lung is cancerous, a **lobectomy** can remove a single, specific lobe of the lung. A **bilobectomy** is the removal of two lobes.

What are the bronchioles? What are the alveolar ducts and sacs? What are the pulmonary alveoli?

Distal to the tertiary (or segmental) bronchi are the **bronchioles.** This final aspect of the **conducting zone** (i.e., the nose, pharynx, larynx, trachea, bronchi, and bronchioles) consists of both terminal and respiratory bronchioles. Twenty to twenty-five **terminal bronchioles** branch directly from each tertiary bronchi. Club cells in the terminal bronchioles secrete surfactant to help provide patency during ventilation. The **respiratory bronchioles** have connections from each terminal bronchiole to the **alveolar ducts**. Each alveolar duct continues to 5–6 **alveolar sac** clusters, which resemble a cluster of grapes. Within each alveolar sac, individual **pulmonary alveolus** (like one grape within a cluster of grapes) provide the functional unit of gas exchange. Each alveolus is surrounded by an **alveolar capillary plexus** within the alveolar wall to enable delivery of deoxygenated blood and removal of re-oxygenated blood.

How is blood re-oxygenated in the pulmonary circulation? How is deoxygenated blood returned to the heart? What vessels supply and drain the lung tissue itself?

Pulmonary circulation re-oxygenates blood via the lungs. The pulmonary trunk bifurcates at the level of T4–T5 IV disc (or the transverse thoracic plane) into a right and a left **pulmonary artery (see figure 6-3A)**. These

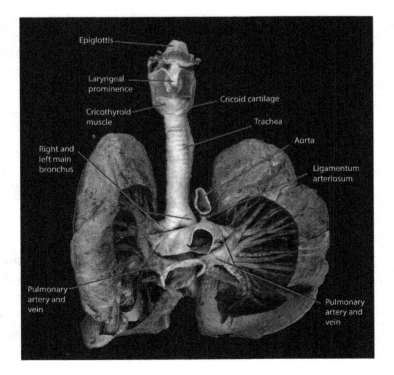

Figure 6-3A

Epiglottis

Laryngeal prominence

Cricothyroid muscle

Cricoid cartilage

Trachea

Aorta

Right and left main bronchus

Ligamentum arteriosum

Pulmonary artery and vein

Pulmonary artery and vein

arteries carry de-oxygenated blood leaving the right ventricle of the heart to the right and left lungs respectively. Because the left lung is closer to the heart, it is shorter than the right pulmonary artery. The right pulmonary artery is located posterior to the ascending aorta. Oxygenation occurs at the alveolar capillary plexus in the alveolar wall and blood is then returned to the left atrium of the heart via the right and left **pulmonary veins (**2–3 on each side; **see figure 6-3A)**. The lung tissue itself receives oxygenated blood through **bronchial arteries** that originate at the aorta**,** and deoxygenated blood drains via the **bronchial veins** into the **azygous system.**

What is the ductus arteriosum? What is the ligamentum arteriosum? What is the patent ductus arteriosum?

A developing fetus (in utero) does not require functioning lungs since oxygen is provided by the mother. Thus, a majority of the blood traveling out of the right ventricle is shunted from the pulmonary trunk to the aortic arch via the **ductus arteriosum**. It includes a short connecting vessel to shunt deoxygenated blood, effectively bypassing the pulmonary circulation and lungs. However, a newborn will initiate breathing immediately after birth, requiring pulmonary function. Thus, the ductus arteriosum normally closes after birth and produces the adult remnant called the **ligamentum arteriosum**. Less frequently, the ductus arteriosum fails to close after birth. This congenital defect, called **patent ductus arteriosum**, impairs oxygenation of blood. Symptoms include shortness of breath and quick fatigue of the infant. If large enough, a patent ductus arteriosum may require corrective surgery.

What impressions are observed on the mediastinal surface of the lungs?

The mediastinal surface (medial aspect) of the lungs has several surface anatomical impressions. On the right lung these include the following: (1) a cardiac impression (inferior), (2) a groove for the esophagus (posterior), (3) the right brachiocephalic vein (superior), (4) the superior vena cava (superior), and (5) a groove for azygous vein. The left lung has similar impressions including (1) a cardiac impression (inferior), (2) a groove for aortic arch and descending aorta (superior, inferior), (3) a groove for esophagus (superior), and (4) a groove for left brachiocephalic vein (superior).

What is a pulmonary embolism?

A pulmonary embolism is when a blood clot becomes lodged or embedded in the pulmonary circulation, which can occlude (or block) blood flow to a specific region (e.g., a lobe or bronchopulmonary segment). Patients frequently experience shortness of breath and difficulty breathing, or even rare sudden death. Deep vein thrombosis (i.e, a blood clot) of the lower limb or pelvic region account for 90% of pulmonary embolisms. An example pathway for a pulmonary embolism proceeds through the following structures: (1) blood clot from femoral vein (i.e., the thigh) breaks away, (2) inferior vena cava, (3) right atrium, (4) right atrioventricular valve, (5) right ventricle, (6) pulmonary trunk, (7) right pulmonary artery, (8) pulmonary circulation, (9) blockade of small artery, (10) deprivation of blood to downstream tissue. The mechanism for the release of the thrombus has not elucidated.

How is lymphatic fluid drained from the right and left lungs?

Lymphatic fluid drains from the lungs medially and superiorly. For all lobes of the right lung, the pathway of drainage courses through the following lymph nodes: (1) pulmonary, (2) bronchopulmonary (hilar), (3) inferior tracheobronchial (carinal), (4) right superior tracheobronchial, (5) right paratracheal, to the right bronchomediastinal lymphatic trunk, and ultimately into the right brachiocephalic vein. The drainage pathway for the left lung differs between the superior and inferior lobes. The superior left lobe drainage includes (1) pulmonary, (2) bronchopulmonary (hilar), (3) inferior tracheobronchial (carinal), (4) left superior tracheobronchial, (5) left paratracheal, (6) left bronchomediastinal lymphatic trunk, and (7) left brachiocephalic vein. Lymphatic fluid from the inferior left lobe initially drains similar to the superior left lobe (steps 1–3) but thereafter passes through the (4) right superior tracheobronchial nodes, (5) right paratracheal nodes, into the right bronchomediastinal lymphatic trunk, and finally into right brachiocephalic vein.

See CM 6-3A, 6-3B, and 6-3C for Review.

CM 6-3A

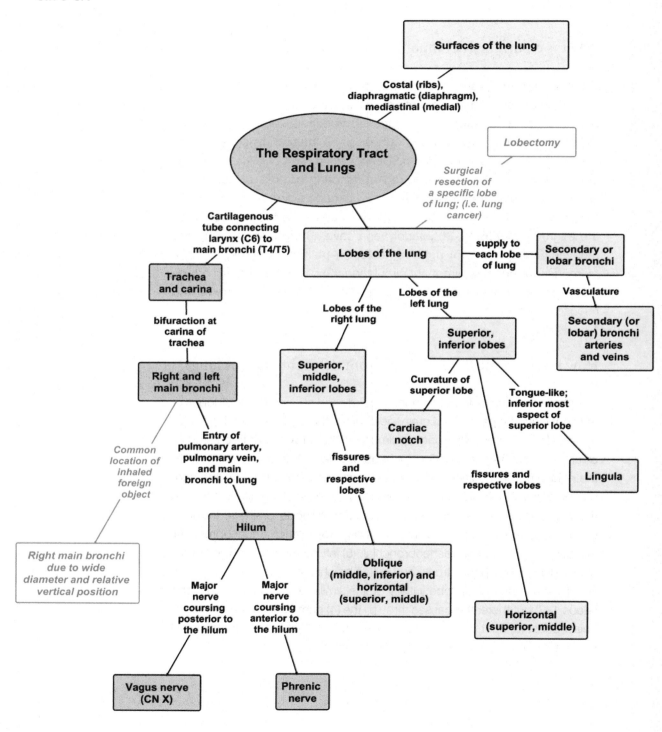

CM 6-3B

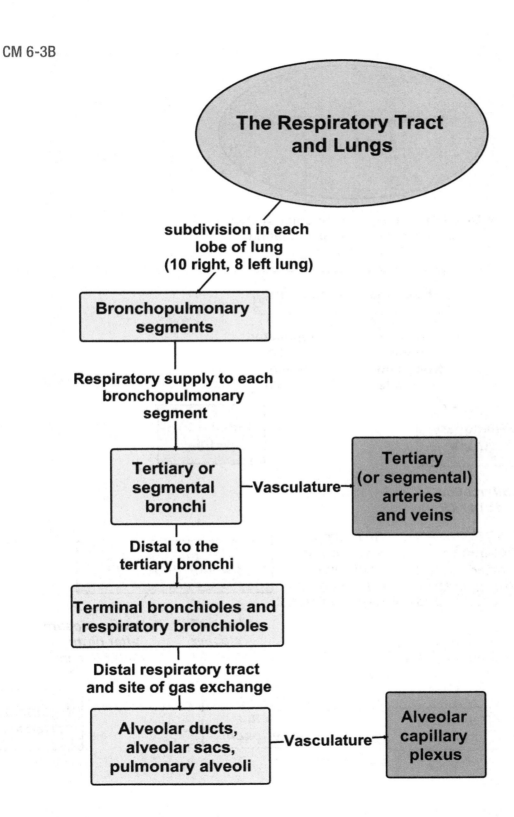

CM 6-3C

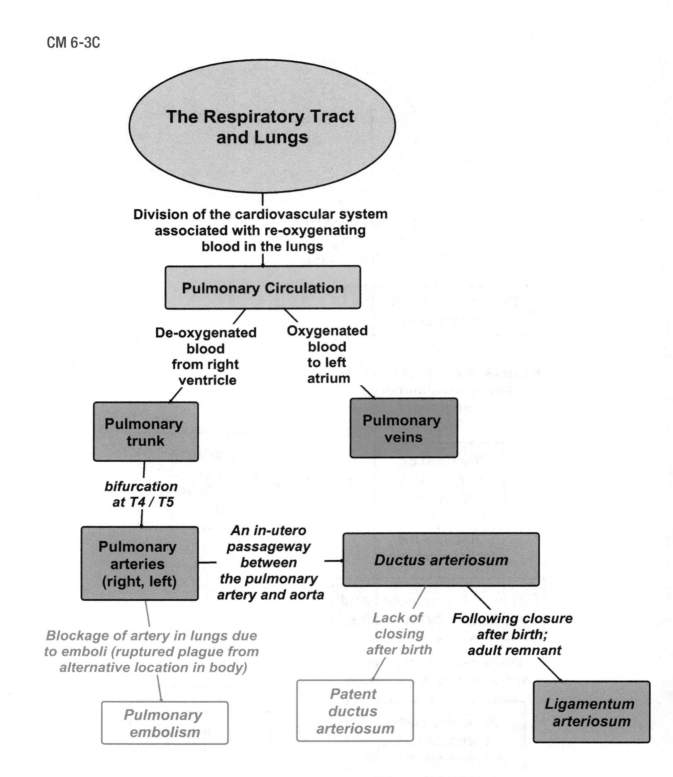

Synthesis Exercise: Create a concept map using items from EXERCISE 6-3A, 6-3B, and 6-3C.

Exercise 6-3A

Primary Category	Secondary Categories	Continuations	Clinical Considerations
Respiratory Tract and Lungs	Surfaces of the lungs Trachea and carina Lobes of the lung	Right and left main bronchi Superior, middle, and inferior lobes Superior and inferior lobes Hilum Cardiac notch Lingula Vagus nerve (CN X) Phrenic nerve Oblique (middle, inferior) and horizontal (superior, middle) Horizontal (superior, middle) Secondary (or lobar) bronchi Secondary (or lobar) arteries and veins	Lobectomy Right main bronchi due to wide diameter and relative vertical position

Exercise 6-3B

Primary Category	Continuations
Respiratory Tract and Lungs	Bronchopulmonary segments Tertiary (or segmental) bronchi Terminal bronchioles and respiratory bronchioles Alvolar ducts, alveolar sacs, and pulmonary alveoli Tertiary (or segmental bronchi) arteries and veins Alveolar capillary plexus

Exercise 6-3C

Primary Category	Secondary Categories	Continuations	Clinical Considerations
Respiratory Tract and Lungs	Pulmonary circulation	Pulmonary trunk Pulmonary veins Pulmonary arteries (right and left) Ductus arteriosus	Pulmonary embolism Patent ductus arteriosum

IV. The Mediastinum

Overview of key topics for this section:

- Location of the mediastinum in the thorax
- Divisions and sub-divisions
- Boundaries and borders
- Contents
- Congenital variations of the aortic arch

Where is the mediastinum? How is it primarily divided? Sub-divided? What are the boundaries and borders of each primary division? What are the contents of each subdivision?

Mediastinum means to *stand in the middle*. This description appropriately defines the centrally placed mediastinum of the thorax, which resides between the right and left pleural cavities. It can be sub-divided into two main divisions, a superior and an inferior mediastinum. The designated border for separation of the two occurs at the transverse thoracic plane (T4/T5 IV disc to sternal angle). Above this plane is the superior mediastinum and below is the inferior mediastinum. Boundaries of the superior mediastinum include the following: (1) superior thoracic aperture (superior border), (2) transverse thoracic plane (inferior border), (3) manubrium (anterior border), (4) T1-T4 vertebral bodies (posterior border), and (5) upper ribs (lateral border). The inferior mediastinum is bound by the following: (1) transverse thoracic plane superior border), (2) diaphragm (inferior border), (3) anterior thoracic wall (anterior border), (4) posterior thoracic wall and vertebral column (posterior border).

Contents of the superior mediastinum include the following: (1) brachiocephalic veins , (2) thoracic duct (3) aortic arch and its branches, (4) major nerves, (5) trachea, and (6) esophagus. The right and left **brachiocephalic veins** (BCV) drain deoxygenated blood into the **superior vena cava,** where it enters the right atrium. Each of the BCVs receive blood from the subclavian vein (drains the upper limb) and the internal jugular vein (drains the head). These veins meet at the right and left **venous angles** and the majority of lymphatic fluid returns to the general circulation at this location. The right

Figure 6-3B

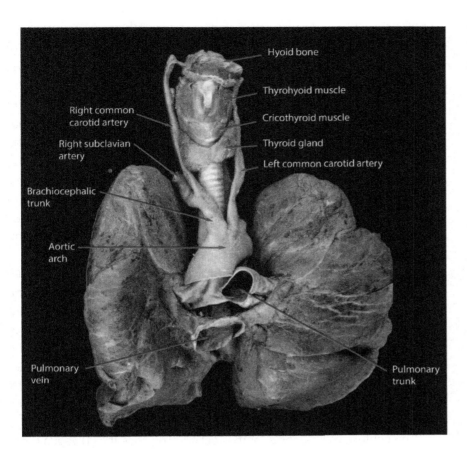

Hyoid bone

Thyrohyoid muscle

Right common
carotid artery

Cricothyroid muscle

Right subclavian
artery

Thyroid gland

Left common carotid artery

Brachiocephalic
trunk

Aortic
arch

Pulmonary
vein

Pulmonary
trunk

venous angle receives lymphatic fluid via the **right lymphatic duct** and the left venous angle collects via the **thoracic duct (see figure 6-2)**. The **aortic arch** of the superior mediastinum carries oxygenated blood from the left ventricle to the systemic circulation. It begins and ends at the transverse thoracic plane by arching superiorly and then inferiorly **(see figure 6-3B)**. It also courses posterior to the left hilum of the lung. The bilateral carotid arteries arise from the proximal aorta and will be described later (see Heart section). The superior aspect of the aortic arch normally gives rise to the brachiocephalic, the left common carotid, and the left subclavian arteries. However, some variation to this pattern can occur. The **brachiocephalic artery** bifurcates into the right subclavian (supplies the right upper limb) and right common carotid artery (supplies the right aspect of the head). The left upper limb and left aspect of the head are supplied by the **left subclavian** and **left common carotid** artery, respectively. Major nerves in the superior mediastinum include the phrenic and vagus nerves. The bilateral phrenic nerve is the sole innervation to the diaphragm and passes anterior to the hilum of the lungs. It also carries sensory information to the pericardium (i.e., sac of the heart), the mediastinal pleura, the diaphragm, and some of the most superior abdominal peritoneum. The right phrenic nerve passes through the diaphragm at the caval foramen (T8 vertebra level) with the inferior vena cava. The left phrenic nerve directly pierces the diaphragm. The bilateral vagus nerve (CN X) branches into the **recurrent laryngeal nerve** (right and left). The right recurrent laryngeal wraps underneath the right subclavian artery to reverse its course towards the larynx, and the left recurrent passes underneath the aortic arch in a similar path. Additional branching of the vagus nerve in the superior mediastinum contributes to the cardiac and pulmonary plexuses. This network of nerves provides their respective organs with parasympathetic innervation. The trachea and esophagus also course through the superior mediastinum.

The inferior mediastinum is further sub-divided into the anterior, middle, and posterior mediastinum. A useful landmark is the **middle mediastinum,** which includes the pericardium (i.e., sac), neurovasculature, and the heart. The anterior mediastinum lies anterior to the pericardium and posterior to the body of the sternum. The **posterior mediastinum** is located posterior to the pericardium and part of the dome-shaped diaphragm; the posterior boundary is the vertebral column (T5–T12). Parietal pleurae of the pleural cavities form the lateral boundaries in each of these sub-divisions for the inferior mediastinum.

The contents of the posterior mediastinum includes the (1) vagus nerve (CN X; right and left), (2) thoracic aorta (descending aorta), (3) esophagus, (4) thoracic duct, (5) azygous venous system, and (6) sympathetic trunk. As the **vagus nerve** courses behind the left and right hilum of the lung, it enters the posterior mediastinum. Branches of the vagus nerve form the esophageal plexus and stimulate waves of smooth muscle contractions (i.e., peristalsis) for the inferior two thirds of the esophagus. It also relaxes the lower esophageal sphincter just prior to a food bolus moving into the stomach. The vagus nerves (or vagal trunks) courses through the diaphragm at the **esophageal hiatus** (T10 vertebral level). The right vagal trunk resides posterior to the esophagus and the left vagal trunk resides anterior to the esophagus.

The **thoracic aorta** (i.e., descending aorta) transports oxygenated blood to the lower half of the body. It resides just to the left of the thoracic vertebra (T5–T12). Several bilateral posterior intercostal arteries branch from the thoracic aorta to supply the intercostal spaces. At the T12 vertebra, the aorta courses through the diaphragm via a passageway called the **aortic**

hiatus and enters the abdominal cavity. Its name appropriately changes to the abdominal aorta.

The **esophagus** is a muscular tube spanning C6–T10 vertebrae and works to transport a food bolus from the laryngopharynx to the stomach. Normal (non-pathologic) constrictions of the esophagus occur at three locations. The laryngopharynx gives rise to the beginning of the esophagus and creates the first constriction. A second constriction is found where the aortic arch and left main bronchi cross anterior to the esophagus. The third constriction occurs at the **esophageal hiatus**, a site where the esophagus passes through the diaphragm (T10 vertebra). Blood supply to the esophagus is via the inferior thyroid artery, bronchial arteries, esophageal arteries, left gastric artery, and the inferior phrenic artery.

The **thoracic duct** is a lymphatic vessel that returns lymphatic fluid from the lower aspect of the body to the left venous angle. Originating in the upper abdominal cavity as the **chyle cistern**, the thoracic duct passes through the diaphragm at the aortic hiatus (T12 vertebra) with the aorta. Negative intrathoracic pressure created during breathing and unidirectional valves help promote return of lymph fluid to the superior aspect of the body through the thoracic duct.

The **azygos vein** drains the posterior thoracic wall into the superior vena cava **(see figure 6-2)**. The left intercostal veins of T5–T8 return blood to the **accessory hemiazygos vein,** which crosses over the T7/T8 vertebra to join the azygos vein on the right side of the posterior mediastinum. The left intercostal veins of T9–T12 drain blood to the **hemiazygos vein** and crosses the T8/T9 vertebrae to also meet the azygos vein. Variation is common among these veins. The right intercostal veins drain directly into the azygos vein and ascends to the superior vena cava. This venous pathway creates an arch similar to the left-sided aortic arch, but the azygos vein courses on the right side. It can be easily observed curving over the right main bronchus of the lung.

Near the left and right sides of the vertebral column, the sympathetic trunk is located within the posterior mediastinum. Thoracic spinal nerves are connected to the sympathetic trunk via white and grey **rami communicans**. This relationship allows connections between the intercostal nerves and the autonomic nervous system. Both cardiopulmonary and abdominopelvic **splanchnic nerves** arise from the sympathetic trunk in this region.

The **anterior mediastinum** is a small area located between the middle mediastinum (pericardium, heart) and the deep aspect of the anterior thoracic wall. The **thymus gland** resides here in children, but begins to atrophy in early teen years. It is a type of specialized lymphoid tissue where maturing lymphocytes, specifically T cells, serve to develop the adaptive immune system. Only remnants of the thymus gland are typically observed in the adult. Also within the anterior mediastinum are the internal thoracic vessels. The **internal thoracic arteries,** or mammary arteries, arise from the subclavian artery and descend deep and lateral to the sternum. The **internal intercostal veins** couple with the arteries and help drain the anterior thoracic wall into the brachiocephalic veins. (Details provided earlier in this chapter.) The **middle mediastinum,** a division of the inferior mediastinum, primarily houses the heart. The next section highlights the heart and its associated structures.

What are the possible congenital variations of the aortic arch?

The aortic arch may vary with regard to some of its major branches as well as its course through the superior mediastinum. The most common pattern of branching (in approximately 65% of the population) proximally to distally includes: (1) the brachiocephalic trunk, branching to the right subclavian and right carotid artery; (2) the left carotid artery; (3) and the left subclavian artery. Smaller percentages of the population have congenital variations that are clinically important for cardiothoracic surgeons. These can include the following patterns from proximal to distal: **Variation A**: (1) Brachiocephalic trunk branching to the right subclavian, right common carotid, and the left common carotid artery, and (2) the left subclavian artery; **Variation B**: (1) Brachiocephalic trunk branching to the right subclavian and right carotid artery, (2) the left carotid artery, (3) left vertebral artery, (4) and the left subclavian artery; **Variation C:** (1) Right brachiocephalic trunk branching to a right subclavian artery and right common carotid artery, and (2) A left brachiocephalic trunk branching to a left subclavian artery and left common carotid artery. Additional branching related variations not listed above may also occur.

The aortic arch may also vary its pathway through the superior mediastinum. For example, a right sided aortic arch can course over the right hilum instead of the left hilum. This variation does not typically produce any impairments. However, a double aortic arch can occur whereby a right and left aorta course around the esophagus and trachea. This rare pattern can lead to compression of the esophagus, trachea, or both.

See CM 6-4A for Review.

CM 6-4A

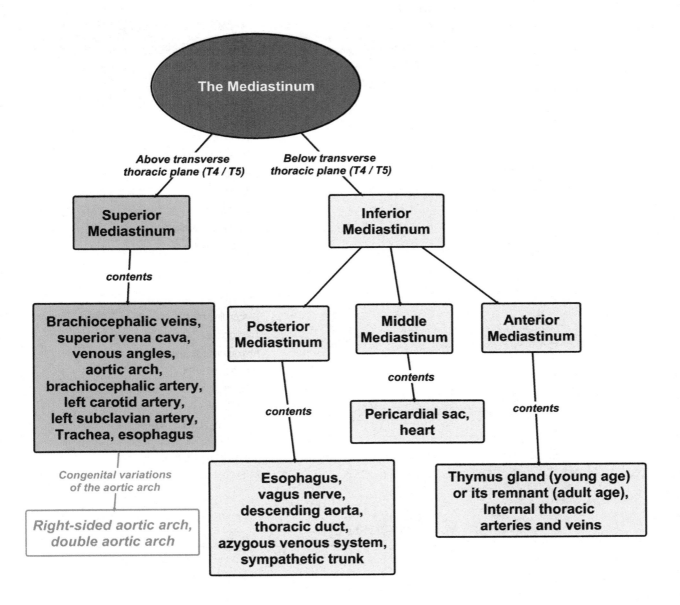

The Mediastinum

Above transverse thoracic plane (T4 / T5)

Below transverse thoracic plane (T4 / T5)

Superior Mediastinum

contents

Brachiocephalic veins, superior vena cava, venous angles, aortic arch, brachiocephalic artery, left carotid artery, left subclavian artery, Trachea, esophagus

Congenital variations of the aortic arch

Right-sided aortic arch, double aortic arch

Inferior Mediastinum

Posterior Mediastinum

Middle Mediastinum

contents

Pericardial sac, heart

contents

Esophagus, vagus nerve, descending aorta, thoracic duct, azygous venous system, sympathetic trunk

Anterior Mediastinum

contents

Thymus gland (young age) or its remnant (adult age), Internal thoracic arteries and veins

Synthesis Exercise: Create a concept map using items from EXERCISE 6-4.

Exercise 6-4

Primary Category	Secondary Categories	Continuations	Clinical Considerations
The mediastinum	Superior mediastinum	Brachiocephalic veins	Right-sided aortic arch,
	Inferior mediastinum	Superior vena cava	Double aortic arch
		Venous angles	
		Aortic arch	
		Brachiocephalic artery	
		Left carotid artery	
		Left subclavian artery	
		Trachea	
		Esophagus	
		Posterior mediastinum	
		Middle mediastinum	
		Anterior mediastinum	
		Esophagus	
		Vagus nerve	
		Descending aorta	
		Thoracic duct	
		Azygous venous system	
		Sympathetic trunk	
		Pericardial Sac	
		Heart	
		Thymus gland (young age) or its remnant (adult age)	
		Internal thoracic arteries and veins	

V. The Heart

Overview of key topics for this section:

- Basic structure and function of the heart
- Heart failure
- The pericardium
- Cardiac tamponade

- Gross anatomy of the heart
- Fetal versus adult circulation
- Coronary vasculature
- The conducting system
- Atherosclerosis
- Coronary artery disease, angioplasty, bypass surgery
- Referred pain

What is the basic structure of the heart? What is the basic function of the heart? What is heart failure?

The heart is a four chambered organ located in the middle mediastinum of the thorax. It includes a right atrium, right ventricle, left atrium, and left ventricle. Blood is pumped through each chamber via a series of cardiac muscle contractions called **systole**, and relaxations called **diastole**. On the right side of the heart, deoxygenated blood is pumped to the lungs for re-oxygenation, a process termed **pulmonary circulation**. On the left side, oxygenated blood is pumped to all parts of the body except the lungs (i.e., **systemic circulation**). On a cellular level, the heart consists primarily of cardiac myocytes, which produce force during systole and relaxation during diastole. A single cardiac cycle is one part systole and one part diastole. Each minute the heart typically repeats about 70 cardiac cycles at rest (i.e., 70 beats per minute; or 70 bpm). In response to metabolic flux (e.g., exercise), the heart can significantly change the number of cardiac cycles from 70 to 200 per minute. **Heart failure** refers to the inability of the heart to meet the metabolic demands of the body. This important clinical concept will be discussed later with regard to relevant anatomy of the heart.

What is the pericardium? What is pericardial fluid? What is the epicardium?

The pericardium, or pericardial sac, is a fibro-serous sac that surrounds the heart. The sac is characterized as having two main parts, one fibrous and one serous. The external layer is the **fibrous pericardium,** composed of dense, loose, connective tissues. The **serous pericardium** resides internally and specialized cells secrete pericardial fluid in the sac as a lubricant. The **serous parietal pericardium** is located on the internal lining of the fibrous pericardium, and the **serous visceral pericardium** actually lines the heart itself (i.e., **epicardium**). Between these two layers lies the pericardial cavity, which houses pericardial fluid. The **pericardiacophrenic artery** supplies the pericardium, which is innervated by the **phrenic nerve**.

What is cardiac tamponade? What is pericardiocentesis?

Fluid can accumulate inside the pericardial cavity (or pericardial effusion). A limited amount of pericardial fluid is not harmful to the performance of the heart, but excessive fluid buildup can lead to **cardiac tamponade**. In this condition, the fluid inside the pericardial sac leads to increased intrapericardial pressure, compressing the heart. Cardiac tamponade typically impairs normal performance of the heart and a patient may require **pericardiocentesis**, a procedure that removes excessive pericardial fluid. A clinician inserts a needle into the pericardial sac at two common locations, the infrasternal angle, or through the fifth or sixth intercostal space near the left border of the sternum.

What are the gross external features of the heart?

The superior aspect of the heart, known as the **base**, is identified by several major vessels exiting the heart. The most inferior aspect of the heart has a roundish feature called the **apex (see figure 6-4A)**. The heart's apex is typically positioned more leftward in the thorax rather than directly midline. However, during deep inspiration the apex pulls inferiorly and more vertically as a result of its attachment to the diaphragm. Thus, the heart's position is considered to be dynamic, which becomes important during imaging and techniques such as pericardiocentesis. Anteriorly, the pulmonary trunk exits the right ventricle at the heart's base. The aortic arch exits the left ventricle, but its proximal end is located just to the right of the pulmonary trunk. The inferior vena cava (IVC) and superior vena cava (SVC) on the right side of the heart in the posterior view; both of these major veins deliver deoxygenated blood to the right atrium. Pulmonary veins (usually 2–3 on each side) are located on the posterior surface near the heart's base. The auricles of the right and left atrium are also typically the base, and are described as resembling dog-like ears. A passageway known as the **transverse sinus**

Figure 6-4A

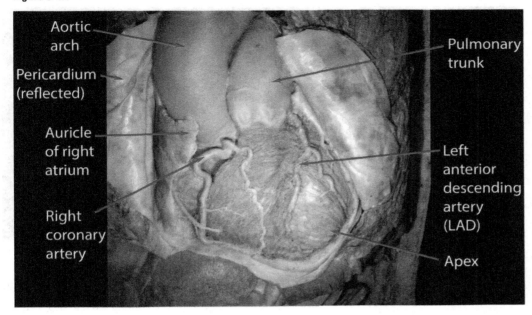

Aortic arch

Pericardium (reflected)

Auricle of right atrium

Right coronary artery

Pulmonary trunk

Left anterior descending artery (LAD)

Apex

sits posterior to the pulmonary trunk and ascending aorta. The **oblique sinus** is a partially enclosed space posterior to heart. The internal gross anatomy of the heart will be described next.

What are the gross internal features of the heart? What is the myocardium? Endocardium?

The internal chambers of the heart are partially separated via walls of cardiac tissue called septa. The division between the right and left atrium is called the **interatrial septum,** and separation of the ventricles is due to the **interventricular septum.** Several valves also help separate atria and ventricles on each side of the heart. Together, the internal heart has a total of four chambers. The two atria (superior) are smaller chambers than the larger ventricles (inferior). Size and location of each chamber help with identification of the major vessels and internal anatomy of the heart.

The right side of the heart pumps deoxygenated blood to the lungs, or pulmonary circulation. Within the **right atrium**, **pectinate muscles** appear as multiple ridges of muscle fibers near the anterior aspect of this chamber

Figure 6-4B

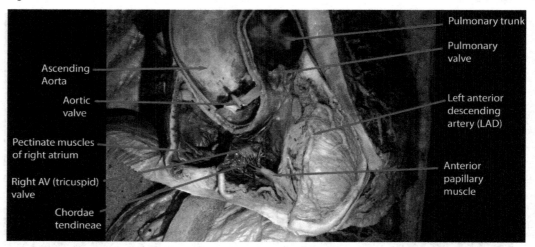

Ascending Aorta

Aortic valve

Pectinate muscles of right atrium

Right AV (tricuspid) valve

Chordae tendineae

Pulmonary trunk

Pulmonary valve

Left anterior descending artery (LAD)

Anterior papillary muscle

(see figure 6-4B). The **crista terminalis** is a transition from the pectinate muscles to the smooth posterior wall. An adult remnant of embryological development in the heart called the **fossa oval,** is located on the interatrial wall (see next section for more detail). In addition to the venous openings of the IVC and SVC, deoxygenated coronary blood is delivered to the right atrium via the **opening of the coronary sinus**. The right atrium pumps blood into the right ventricle via the **right atrioventricular valve** (right AV valve, or tricuspid valve). This valve has three cusps including the anterior, posterior, and septal cusps. Each cusp attaches to **papillary muscles** of the right ventricular wall or septum via **chordae tendinae** (tendinous chords). At the beginning of systole, the papillary muscles contract. Chordae tendinae pull the cusps together and help prevent prolapsing into the right atrium. The **septomarginal band (or moderator band)** attaches from the interventricular septa to the chordae tendinae of the anterior cusp. Electrical conduction to, and contraction of, the septomarginal band can occur early in systole as a result of its association with the interventricular septum. Due to increasing intraventricular pressure during systole, blood is ejected out of the right ventricle through the **pulmonary valve** and into the pulmonary trunk **(see figure 6-4C)**. This valve has three semilunar cusps: the anterior, right, and the left cusp. A cone-like space just before passage through the pulmonary valve is called the **conus arteriosus**. The **trabeculae carneae** are muscular ridges on internal surface of ventricular wall.

The left side of the heart pumps blood to the systemic circulation. The **left atrium** is similar to the right. However, pulmonary veins containing

Figure 6-4C

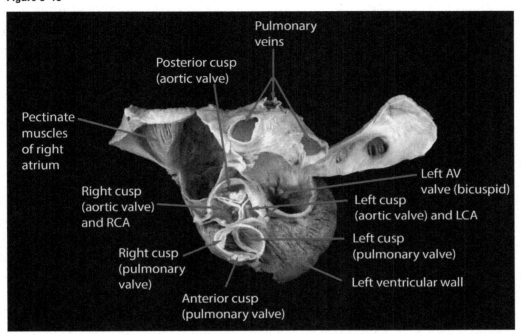

oxygenated blood enter the left atrium. Blood is pumped out of the left atrium into the left ventricle through the **left atrioventricular valve** (left AV valve, bicuspid, or mitral valve). This valve has only 2 cusps including an anterior and a posterior. Similar to the right ventricle, the left ventricle has papillary muscles and chordae tendinae to help close the left AV valve during systole. Trabecular carneae are also found on the internal wall of the left ventricle. At the end of the systole, increased intraventricular pressure in the left ventricle ejects blood into the aorta through the **aortic valve (see figure 6-4D)**. This valve has three semilunar cusps including a right, left, and posterior cusp. **Aortic sinuses** are present during filling of the proximal end of the aorta. These spaces are located between the wall of the proximal aorta and the cusps of the aortic valve. Both coronary arteries (right and left) begin in the aortic sinuses, and, thus, fill with oxygenated blood at the end of systole. Auscultation of valves via a stethoscope is important for di- agnosing valve dysfunction and retrograde blood flow (i.e. a heart murmur). The left ventricular wall is typically much thicker than the right side due to the amount of force required to pump blood through the systemic versus pulmonary circulations. This feature can often help students navigate the major vessels and chambers of the internal heart.

The **myocardium** is just deep to the epicardium, houses the cardiac muscle tissue for contractions. Grossly, it can be observed as the thick aspect of a dissected ventricular wall. The **endocardium** line the chambers of the heart and valves with cells are similar to endothelial cells in blood vessels.

What are key differences between fetal and adult hearts? What congenital heart defects can potentially develop following birth?

Due to the lack of pulmonary function in utero (before birth), the fetal heart has two key differences as compared to an adult. The **foramen ovale** is an opening of the interatrial septum, allowing blood to bypass pulmonary circulation. Since the fetus receives oxygen from mother, blood is not required to circulate the lungs. Thus, blood passes from the right atrium to the left atrium via the foramen ovale. Upon birth, this passageway typically closes and an adult remnant is called the **fossa oval**. However, a patent fossa ovale that does not close can lead to a shortness of breath, fatigue, and heart palpitations. A second conduit i.e., (passageway) to bypass the pulmonary circulation in the fetal heart is the **ductus arteriosum.** It has a small vessel connecting the pulmonary trunk and aorta. Thus, blood that does reach the pulmonary trunk is shunted towards the aorta. After birth, this becomes an adult remnant called the **ligamentum arteriosum.** Similar to a patent fossa ovale, a patent ductus arteriosum can remain open after birth. Surgical intervention is usually required for both types of congenital heart defects.

What provides arterial supply to the heart? What veins drain the heart?

The heart receives oxygenated blood via a collection of branches from the **coronary arteries**. Both the right and left coronary artery help meet the oxygen demands of the heart. Although each coronary artery supplies the respective side of the heart (left versus right), a heart can be considered right-dominant or left-dominant based on which coronary artery is the chief supplier. Which coronary artery supplies the posterior descending artery

Figure 6-4D

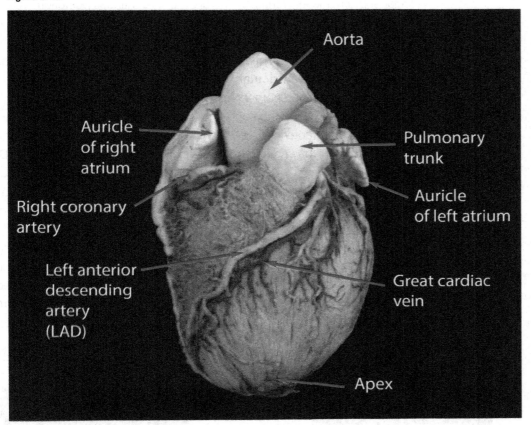

(or posterior interventricular) usually determines which artery is the chief supplier. About 70% of the population is right-dominant.

The **right coronary artery** (RCA) originates from the proximal aorta from within right aortic sinus **(see figure 6-4D)**. It quickly gives rise to a **sinoatrial nodal branch** to supply pacemaker cells within the sinoartial node. The RCA continues within the **atrial-ventricular sulcus**, a groove between the atria and ventricles. On the right and lateral aspect of the heart, a **right marginal branch** supplies the right heart. In the posterior heart, a **posterior interventricular branch** typically arises from the RCA and supplies the posterior aspect of the interventricular septum.

The **left coronary artery** (LCA) also begins from the proximal aorta, but from within the left aortic sinus. Its first branch is the **left anterior descending artery** (LAD, or anterior descending, or anterior interventricular) **(see figure 6-4C)**. The path of the LAD is within the interventricular septum on the anterior surface of the heart and ultimately can anastomose with the posterior descending artery. The LAD serves the anterior interventricular septum and left ventricle. The distal LCA continues posteriorly within the interventricular sulcus as the **left circumflex artery**. On the left and lateral aspect, a **left marginal artery** branches to help supply the left heart. The left circumflex artery continues posteriorly and will occasionally give rise to a **posterior interventricular branch.**

Deoxygenated blood from the myocardium drains via a collection of coronary veins. It returns to the right atrium and flows towards the pulmonary circulation. On the anterior heart, the **great cardiac vein** is located in the interventricular sulcus and parallels the left anterior descending artery (LAD) **(see figure 6-4C)**. On the posterior surface, the **middle cardiac vein** couples with the posterior descending artery within the interventricular sulcus **(see figure 6-4E)**. Both veins drain the anterior and posterior aspects of the heart. The **small cardiac vein,** on the right aspect of the heart, helps drain the right ventricular wall. All of the above vessels drain into a collecting reservoir located posteriorly within the atrioventricular sulcus, called the **coronary sinus (see figure 6-4E)**. Upon collection, blood is returned to the right atrium from the coronary sinus through the **opening of the coronary sinus.**

Figure 6-4E

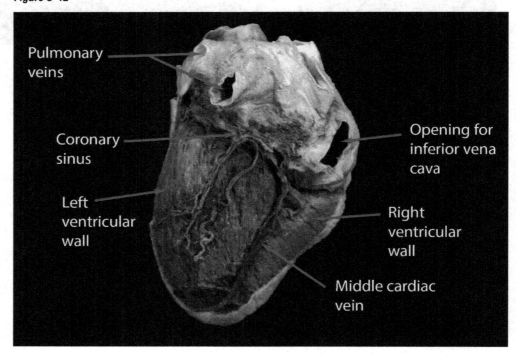

What is atherosclerosis? What risk factors are involved?

Over the course of several years or decades, the lumen of some arteries may narrow (i.e., stenosis) due to the formation of plaque (or atheroma). This disease, called **atherosclerosis,** can affect arteries in the heart, brain, limbs, and other areas. The plaque is composed of foam cells, lipids, and cholesterol. It restricts blow flow to distal tissues such as the myocardium. The mechanism of development is unclear. However, specific risk factors are known to include overnutrition, physical inactivity, and smoking.

What is coronary artery disease? Myocardial infarction?

Atherosclerosis in the heart can promote the development of **coronary artery disease (CAD)**. For example, decreases in blood supply via a coronary artery can lead to impaired cardiac performance. If the atherosclerotic plaque ruptures, an embolism is released and can lodge within a downstream artery. Thus, occluding the supply of oxygen and energy substrates can lead to a **myocardial infarction** (MI, or heart attack). Acute pain in the chest, called **angina,** is a common indication of MI and CAD. Ischemia or lack of sufficient oxygen supply can damage the muscle tissue of the heart (i.e., the myocardium). Common sites of CAD or MI within the coronary arteries include the following: (1) left anterior descending (LAD), (2) right coronary artery, (3) left coronary artery, (4) posterior interventricular artery. Nitroglycerin is a medication used to immediately help treat MI and angina. It is a vasodilator which serves to relieve occlusion of the impacted coronary artery.

What is coronary angioplasty? Coronary artery bypass surgery?

Following the evaluation of coronary blood flow via an **angiogram**, an interventional cardiologist may choose to perform **coronary balloon angioplasty** for a patient with coronary artery disease. This technique introduces a catheter into the femoral artery which is guided into the coronary arterial system. X-ray imaging allows for the specific placement of the catheter near the occluded vessel. The tip of the angioplasty, or balloon, is inflated and thus disrupts the atherosclerotic plague. A **coronary stent** can also be introduced to maintain patency of the vessel. An alternative technique is **coronary bypass surgery**. For example, the internal thoracic artery (thorax; direct attachment) or a portion of the great saphenous vein (thigh; harvested and connected to aorta) can be surgically connected to a coronary artery. This method can effectively bypass blood around an obstructed coronary artery and may include one or more bypasses (a single bypass involves one artery, double bypass involves two arteries, etc.). Both coronary angioplasty and bypass surgery can improve coronary blood flow and myocardial function.

What is referred pain? How does it relate to a myocardial infarction?

Referred pain can be perceived at a location other than the origin of the pain stimulus. For example, dying or damaged cardiac myocytes will communicate pain to the spinal cord and brain via general visceral afferent nerve fibers. However, somatic afferent nerve fibers from T1–T4, that supply the left thorax and left upper limb, follow the same pathway as the heart. Thus, the central nervous system cannot clearly distinguish between visceral and somatic nerve impulses (e.g., pain). A common indication of a myocardial infarction is angina (chest pain or discomfort) often with numbness of the left shoulder and left upper limb.

What system communicates the heart to contract?

The **conducting system of the heart** is composed of cardiac pacemaker cells called nodes (or group), cardiac myocytes, and conducting fibers. Each component works to transmit, or spread, electrical signals called **action potentials** to stimulate a cardiac contraction. The action potentials originate in a collection of specialized pacemaker cells in the upper right atrium, called the **sinoatrial node (SA node)**. It sets the overall pace of the cardiac cycle and is influenced by innervation (e.g., sympathetic, vagus nerves) and hormones (e.g., epinephrine, norepinephrine). The action potentials are conveyed (i.e., spread) through the atrium via gap junctions in the cardiac myocytes. This signals the atrium to contract. A secondary set of specialized pacemaker cells, the **atrioventricular node (AV node)**, is located in the lower right atrium near the heart's midline. The atrium receives action potentials at this location conveys them through the interventricular septum (superior to inferior) via conducting fibers. The **atrioventricular (AV) bundle** propagates the action potentials from the AV node to the most superior aspect of the septum. The bundle bifurcates into the **right and left bundle branches** to span the remaining interventricular septum. The distal aspect of the conduction system begins near the apex and includes the subendocardial branches (**Purkinje fibers**). Multiple subendocardial branches invest into the right and left ventricular walls. Finally, the action potentials reach the ventricular walls and facilitate a contraction.

See CM 6-5A, 6-5B, 6-5C, 6-5D, and 6-5E for Review.

CM 6-5A

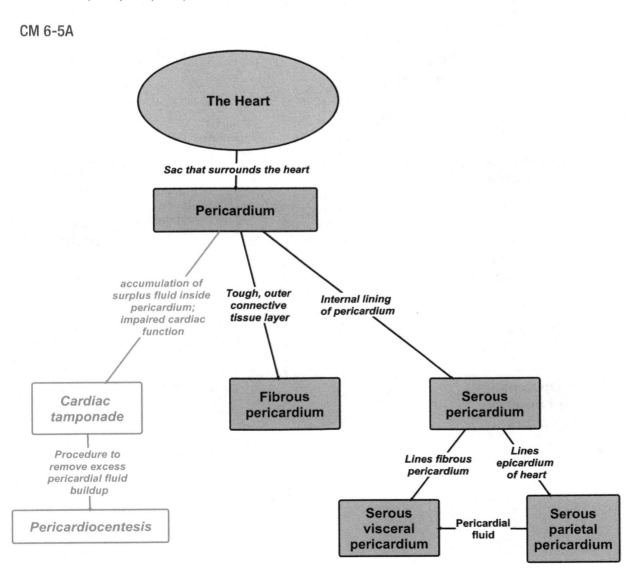

CM 6-5B

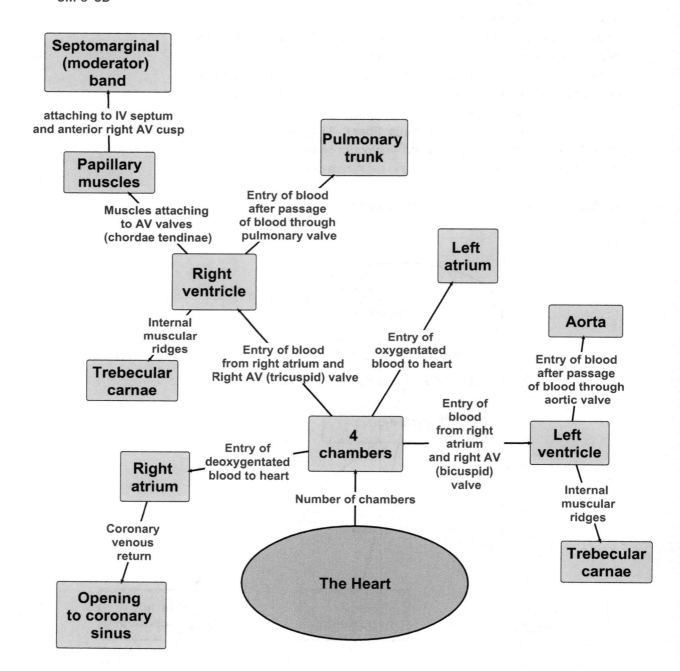

Septomarginal (moderator) band

attaching to IV septum and anterior right AV cusp

Papillary muscles

Muscles attaching to AV valves (chordae tendinae)

Pulmonary trunk

Entry of blood after passage of blood through pulmonary valve

Left atrium

Right ventricle

Internal muscular ridges

Entry of oxygentated blood to heart

Aorta

Entry of blood after passage of blood through aortic valve

Trebecular carnae

Entry of blood from right atrium and Right AV (tricuspid) valve

4 chambers

Entry of blood from right atrium and right AV (bicuspid) valve

Left ventricle

Entry of deoxygentated blood to heart

Internal muscular ridges

Right atrium

Number of chambers

Coronary venous return

The Heart

Trebecular carnae

Opening to coronary sinus

CM 6-5C

CM 6-5D

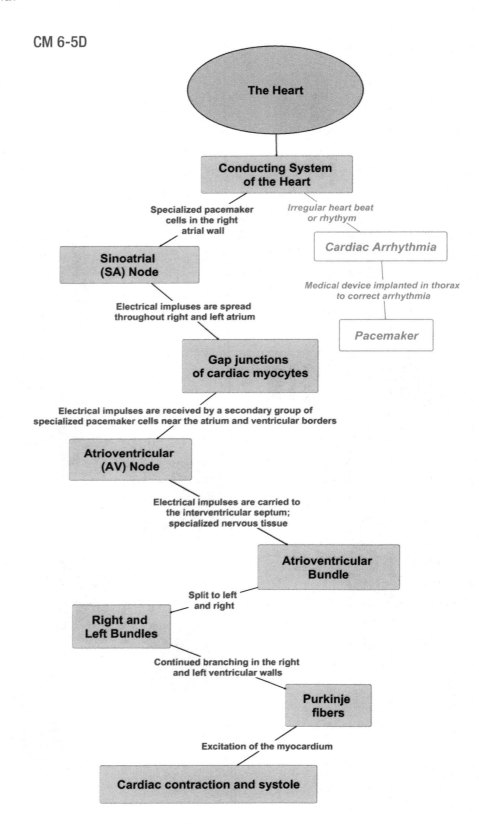

CM 6-5E

The Heart

Structural impairments of the heart at birth

Congenital heart defects

Foramen ovale fails to close after birth allowing blood to bypass pulmonary circulation; Blood is not fully oxygenated

Patent foramen ovale

Narrowing or hardening of coronary blood vessel lumen due to atherosclerosis; can lead to ischemia of the heart

Coronary artery disease

Actue blockade of a coronary vessel by a rupture of atherosclerotic plaque

Myocardial Infarction (MI)

Pain at an location different than the site of pain stimulus; Example- during MI, a patient also perceives numbness in the left upper limb

Referred pain

Inability of the heart to meet the metabolic demands of the body

Heart failure

Narrowing of blood vessel lumen due to plaque formation

Atheroslcerosis

Invasive surgery to ligate new vessel around a blocked coronary artery ("bypass")

Coronary bypass surgery

Minimally invasive procedure used to widen a narrow coronary artery by inflating a balloon; a vascular stent may also be left in place to maintain patency

Coronary angioplasty

CHAPTER 6

Synthesis Exercise: Create a concept map using items from EXERCISE 6-5A, 6-5B, 6-5C, 6-5D, and 6-5E.

Exercise 6-5A

Primary Category	Secondary Categories	Continuations	Clinical Considerations
The heart	Pericardium	Fibrous pericardium	Cardiac tamponade
		Serous pericardium	Pericardiocentesis
		Serous visceral pericardium	
		Serous parietal pericardium	

Exercise 6-5B

Primary Category	Secondary Categories	Continuations
The heart	4 chambers	Right atrium
		Right ventricle
		Left atrium
		Left ventricle
		Opening to coronary sinus
		Trabeculae carnae
		Papillary muscles
		Septomarginal (moderator) band
		Pulmonary trunk
		Aorta
		Trabeculae carnae

Exercise 6-5C

Primary Category	Secondary Categories	Continuations
The heart	Coronary arterial system	Right coronary artery (RCA)
	Coronary venous system	Left coronary artery (LCA)
		SA nodal branch
		Right marginal branch
		Posterior interventricular
		Left anterior descending (LAD)
		Left marginal branch
		Circumflex branch
		Coronary sinus
		Small cardiac vein
		Middle cardiac vein
		Great cardiac vein

Exercise 6-5D

Primary Category	Secondary Categories	Continuations	Clinical Considerations
The heart	Conducting system of the heart	Sinoatrial (SA) node	Cardiac arrhythmia
		Gap junctions of cardiac myocytes	Pacemaker
		Atrioventricular (AV) node	
		Atrioventricular bundle	
		Right and left bundle branches	
		Purkinje fibers	
		Cardiac contraction and systole	

Exercise 6-5E

Primary Category	Clinical Considerations
The heart	Congenital heart defects
	Patent foramen ovale
	Atherosclerosis
	Coronary bypass surgery
	Coronary angioplasty
	Coronary artery disease
	Myocardial infarction (MI)
	Heart failure
	Referred pain

Image Credits

- Fig. 6-1: Copyright © 2017 by 4D Anatomy. Reprinted with permission.
- Fig. 6-2: Copyright © 2017 by 4D Anatomy. Reprinted with permission.
- Fig. 6-3A: Copyright © 2017 by 4D Anatomy. Reprinted with permission.
- Fig. 6-3B: Copyright © 2017 by 4D Anatomy. Reprinted with permission.
- Fig. 6-4A: Copyright © 2017 by 4D Anatomy. Reprinted with permission.
- Fig. 6-4B: Copyright © 2017 by 4D Anatomy. Reprinted with permission.
- Fig. 6-4C: Copyright © 2017 by 4D Anatomy. Reprinted with permission.
- Fig. 6-4D: Copyright © 2017 by 4D Anatomy. Reprinted with permission.
- Fig. 6-4E: Copyright © 2017 by 4D Anatomy. Reprinted with permission

References

Blunt JR, Karpicke JD, J Educational Psychology, 2014 Vol. 106, No. 3, 849–858, "Learning With Retrieval-Based Concept Mapping"

Moore, Keith, Anne M. R. Agur, and Arthur F. Dalley. 2013. *Clinically Oriented Anatomy, 7th ed.*. Baltimore: Lippincott. Williams & Wilkins, 2014.

Moore, Keith, Anne M. R. Agur, and Arthur F. Dalley. 2005. *Essential Clinical Anatomy, 5th ed.*. Baltimore: Lippincott.Williams & Wilkins, 2011.

CPSIA information can be obtained
at www.ICGtesting.com
Printed in the USA
LVOW05s1149231217
560587LV00002B/4/P